50% OFF

Online Cardiac-Vascular Nursing Prep Course!

Dear Customer,

Thank you for your purchase of this Cardiac-Vascular Nursing Study Guide. Included with your purchase is **discounted access to our online Cardiac-Vascular Nursing Prep Course**. Many Cardiac-Vascular Nursing courses are needlessly expensive and don't deliver enough value. Our course provides the best Cardiac-Vascular Nursing prep material, and with discounted access, **you only pay half price**.

We have structured our online course to perfectly complement your printed study guide. The Cardiac-Vascular Nursing Prep Course contains **in-depth lessons** that cover all the most important topics, **450 practice questions** to ensure you feel prepared, and more than **550 digital flashcards**, so you can study while you're on the go.

Online Cardiac-Vascular Nursing Prep Course

Topics Included:

- Assessment and Diagnosis
  - Anatomy, Physiology, and Pathophysiology
  - Patient Interview
- Planning and Implementation
  - Evidence-Based Guidelines and Quality Improvement
  - Scope and Standards of Practice
- Evaluation and Modification
- Patient and Community Education
  - Cardiac-Vascular Risk Factors
  - Education Topics

Course Features:

- Cardiac-Vascular Nursing Study Guide
  - Get content that complements our best-selling study guide.
- Full-Length Practice Tests
  - With 450 practice questions, you can test yourself again and again.
- Mobile Friendly
  - If you need to study on the go, the course is easily accessible from your mobile device.
- Cardiac-Vascular Nursing Flashcards
  - Our course includes a flashcard mode with over 550 content cards to help you study.

To lock in your discounted access, visit mometrix.com/university/cardiacvascular or simply scan this QR code with your smartphone. At the checkout page, enter the discount code: **cvn50off**

If you have any questions or concerns, please contact us at support@mometrix.com.

Mometrix
TEST PREPARATION

AF834535

Cardiac/Vascular Nurse Exam Practice Questions

Mometrix
TEST PREPARATION

Dear Future Exam Success Story

First of all, **THANK YOU** for purchasing Mometrix study materials!

Second, congratulations! You are one of the few determined test-takers who are committed to doing whatever it takes to excel on your exam. **You have come to the right place.** We developed these practice tests with one goal in mind: to deliver you the best possible approximation of the questions you will see on test day.

Standardized testing is one of the biggest obstacles on your road to success, which only increases the importance of doing well in the high-pressure, high-stakes environment of test day. Your results on this test could have a significant impact on your future, and these practice tests will give you the repetitions you need to build your familiarity and confidence with the test content and format to help you achieve your full potential on test day.

Your success is our success

We would love to hear from you! If you would like to share the story of your exam success or if you have any questions or comments in regard to our products, please contact us at **800-673-8175** or **support@mometrix.com**.

Thanks again for your business and we wish you continued success!

Sincerely,
The Mometrix Test Preparation Team

Written and edited by the Mometrix Exam Secrets Test Prep Team
Printed in the United States of America

Table of Contents

Practice Test #1

1. Persistent atrial fibrillation is defined as fibrillation that:

a. Ends spontaneously or with treatment within 1 week
b. Continues for more than 1 week
c. Continues for more than 1 year
d. Cannot be converted to sinus rhythm

2. The PQRST method of angina assessment includes (P) precipitating factors, (Q) quality of pain, (R) radiation of pain, (S) severity of pain, and (T):

a. Trend
b. Tolerance
c. Tiredness
d. Timing

3. When teaching a patient with coronary artery disease to control angina, the first step is to:

a. Determine what precipitates episodes.
b. Stress the importance of taking medications correctly.
c. Encourage patient to maintain a healthy diet.
d. Advise patient to engage in regular exercise to tolerance.

4. Which of the following activities would be classified as a moderate-energy activity (3–6 metabolic equivalents [METs])?

a. Washing the face and hands
b. Ascending a flight of stairs
c. Using a bedside commode
d. Eating

5. If percutaneous coronary intervention (PCI), such as coronary angioplasty, is to be used to treat a patient with an acute MI with an occluded coronary artery, the PCI should be performed within:

a. 10 hours
b. 6 hours
c. 3 hours
d. 90 minutes

6. If telemetry shows a regular heart rate of 64 bpm with normal P wave, normal QRS complex, and PR interval of 0.25 seconds, the heart rhythm would be classified as exhibiting:

a. Normal sinus rhythm
b. First-degree AV block
c. Sinus bradycardia
d. Second-degree AV block, type II

7. A patient who has been hospitalized for heart failure has been encouraged to ambulate and complains of discomfort in the right posterior thigh area with tenderness to palpation but no visible erythema. What change in the plan of care is immediately indicated?

a. Bedrest
b. Fluid restriction
c. Low-sodium diet
d. Physical therapy

8. As part of the US Department of Health and Human Services' 5 A's (ask, advise, assess, assist, and arrange follow-up) guidelines for smoking cessation, during the "assist" stage, patients should be asked to establish a target date for quitting that is within:

a. 4 days
b. 7 days
c. 14 days
d. 21 days

9. The intensity of a heart murmur that is loud and accompanied by a thrill would be classified as grade:

a. I/VI
b. II/VI
c. III/VI
d. IV/VI

10. According to the National Heart, Lung, and Blood Institute Adult Treatment Panel III (ATP III) recommendations for cholesterol management, the primary target of therapy for LDL cholesterol is:

a. <80 mg/dL
b. <100 mg/dL
c. 100–129 mg/dL
d. 130–159 mg/dL

11. Which of the following tests is the best marker for ventricular dysfunction and heart failure?

a. Atrial natriuretic peptide
b. C-reactive protein
c. B-type natriuretic peptide
d. Homocysteine

12. When using the SMART format to develop targeted goals, these goals should be (S) specific, (M) measurable, (A) attainable, (R) realistic, and (T):

a. Timely
b. Temporary
c. Topical
d. Tested

13. When a patient is faced with a serious illness, the most effective initial intervention to assist the patient with coping skills is to:

a. Provide a list of coping strategies.
b. Use a calm and reassuring approach.
c. Ask the patient about past coping behavior.
d. Provide factual information about the disease.

14. The cardiac care supervisor is considering switching from 8-hour work schedules to 12-hour work schedules, with some staff members adamantly in favor and some adamantly opposed. During a meeting called to discuss the issue, the first step in resolving the conflict should be to:

a. Allow both sides to present their opinions.
b. Encourage cooperation.
c. Provide reasons for the change.
d. State that the supervisor will make the decision.

15. Which of the following troponin I levels indicate cardiac injury?

a. <0.04 ng/mL
b. >0.40 ng/mL
c. >4 ng/mL
d. >0.04 ng/mL

16. According to the ACCF/AHA heart failure guideline, the most important intervention for treatment of stage A heart failure is:

a. Reduction in obesity
b. Treatment of dyslipidemia
c. Control of hypertension
d. Control of hyperglycemia

17. In the design of the delivery system under the Chronic Care Model of disease management, patients should be provided care that:

a. Focuses on patient and family needs
b. Focuses on lifestyle changes
c. Is affordable and flexible
d. Is understandable and culturally appropriate

18. When utilizing the $CHADS_2$ stratification score to estimate stroke risk for patients with nonvalvular atrial fibrillation, each increase of 1 point on the scale increases risk of stroke by approximately:

a. 1%
b. 2%
c. 3%
d. 4%

19. Which of the following signs is associated with peripheral venous insufficiency?

a. Pitting edema
b. Rubor on dependency
c. Ulcerations on toes
d. Pale, shiny skin

20. A patient is brought to the ED after collapsing at a public event and is believed to have had a myocardial infarction, but the patient adamantly refuses all care because she is a Christian Scientist. The best response of the nurse is:

a. "You could die without treatment."
b. "Let's talk about lifestyle changes that may help."
c. "Is your religion more important than your life?"
d. "You really need treatment because your heart has been damaged."

21. The key component of health promotion is:

a. Personal responsibility
b. Nutritional awareness
c. Stress reduction techniques/management
d. Physical fitness

22. The cardiac/vascular nurse is demonstrating dressing change procedures to a patient before discharge, but the patient seems confused about the procedure and asks repeatedly, "Can I take notes?" According to VARK classification, the patient's preferred learning style is probably:

a. Visual
b. Aural
c. Read-write
d. Kinesthetic

23. With the ARCS model of motivational design, which aspect focuses on the learner's experience?

a. Attention
b. Relevance
c. Confidence
d. Satisfaction

24. When conducting a motivational interview, the initial assessment should be related to:

a. Cognitive variables
b. Affective variables
c. Physiological variables
d. Environmental variables

25. After completing a dietary assessment with the Fat-Related Diet Habits Questionnaire, the cardiac/vascular nurse asks the patient to maintain a food diary. The optimal period for a food diary is usually:

a. 24 hours
b. 2 days
c. 3 days
d. 1 week

26. When planning an educational program about lifestyle changes for a program of cardiac rehabilitation, the cardiac/vascular nurse recognizes that most adult learners are:

a. Passive
b. Self-directed
c. Unmotivated
d. Anxious

27. When assessing a patient's readiness to learn, which of the following is an aspect of experiential readiness?

a. Developmental stage
b. Task complexity
c. Learning style
d. Previous coping mechanism

28. If a patient with suspected hypertensive crisis presents with BP 200/125 mmHg, the patient's mean arterial pressure (MAP) is:

a. 325 mmHg
b. 75 mmHg
c. 130 mmHg
d. 150 mmHg

29. Which of the following complementary/alternative therapies may decrease LDL, triglycerides, and total cholesterol?

a. Garlic
b. Omega-3 fatty acids
c. Red yeast rice
d. Plant sterols

30. When a patient has an implantable cardioverter-defibrillator, overdrive pacing is utilized for:

a. Ventricular tachycardia
b. Bradycardia
c. Atrial fibrillation
d. Atrial flutter

31. When charged with educating patients about self-care after they have undergone outpatient cardiac procedures, the factor that is most likely to be a barrier to learning is:

a. Patient stress
b. Environment
c. Time constraints
d. Low health literacy

32. When a patient with dilated cardiomyopathy is to be discharged, family members should be advised to:

a. Monitor the patient's medications.
b. Take a CPR course.
c. Avoid leaving the patient alone.
d. Remove all alcohol.

33. Which of the following is an example of a well-written measurable objective?

a. Following three classes, the patient will understand weight-loss principles.
b. The patient will be able to prepare low-calories foods.
c. After self-directed study, the patient will have knowledge of various weight-loss programs and lose weight.
d. Following one-on-one instruction about weight loss, the patient will be able to list four strategies for weight loss.

34. Following a patient's hospitalization for coronary artery bypass grafting (CABG), the primary concern for discharge planning should be:

a. Care and service needs
b. Equipment needs
c. Transportation needs
d. Social needs

35. A 62-year-old male patient with supraventricular tachycardia (SVT) exhibits a pulse rate between 75 and 85 bpm on metoprolol 200 mg daily (100 mg twice daily), but the patient's blood pressure still ranges from 140–150/90–100 mmHg. The risk factor that most needs modification is the patient's:

a. Drinking 2–3 glasses of wine daily
b. Smoking 1 pack of cigarettes daily
c. Walking 30 minutes 4 times weekly
d. Drinking 2 cups of caffeinated tea each morning

36. According to American Heart Association guidelines for exercise, the target heart rate for a patient who is 65 years old and engaging in moderate exercise is:

a. 100–170 bpm
b. 95–162 bpm
c. 90–153 bpm
d. 78–132 bpm

37. A patient with paroxysmal supraventricular tachycardia is to have mobile cardiac event monitoring for a 1-month period with 3 leads connected to a transmitter that sends a message to a cellphone that transmits ECGs to the company. What is the maximum distance that the patient should be from the cellphone?

a. 2 feet
b. 4 feet
c. 6 feet
d. 10 feet

38. The most important factor in interdisciplinary communication is:

a. Clarity
b. Timeliness
c. Respect
d. Knowledge

39. If the cardiac/vascular nurse is interested in advocating for the advancement of nursing practice, the most effective method is to:

a. Network with other nurses in the same field.
b. Write letters to political authorities.
c. Obtain advanced education in the nursing field.
d. Become involved in national organizations.

40. A 58-year-old female patient whose blood pressure had been well controlled during acute and convalescent hospitalization has shown increasing blood pressure readings for the past few weeks since discharge. When questioned about medications, the patient gives vague responses and states, "I have the directions written down at home." The cardiac/vascular nurse should address which of the following potential problems first?

a. Nonadherence
b. Inadequate response to medication
c. Incorrect blood pressure readings
d. Impaired cognitive ability

41. If a patient cannot be weaned off of cardiopulmonary bypass (CPB) after severe acute myocardial injury, the intervention most indicated is:

a. Continued CPB
b. Intra-aortic balloon pump (IABP)
c. Left ventricular assist device (LVAD)
d. Discontinuation of treatments

42. A woman from Saudi Arabia has undergone open-heart surgery and is to return to her country for follow-up treatment but will need wound care and dressing changes. The patient was accompanied by her spouse, children (adolescent daughter and son), and mother. The person to whom the nurse should direct instructions about patient care is the:

a. Spouse
b. Mother
c. Son
d. Daughter

43. A patient has an electrically-powered LVAD with a portable battery pack to use when moving about. If the patient wants to increase activity level, the patient should:

a. Adjust activity to pump speed.
b. Decrease the pump speed.
c. Increase the pump speed.
d. Avoid increasing activity level.

44. A patient who has minimal chest pain on exertion but none at rest and whose coronary angiography shows 90% blockage of the left main coronary artery would be classified according to the NYHA functional classification for heart failure as:

a. Functional capacity 2, objective assessment D
b. Functional capacity 1, objective assessment D
c. Functional capacity 4, objective assessment A
d. Functional capacity 1, objective assessment A

45. Which of the following weight gains may indicate heart failure?

a. 2 pounds in a week
b. 1 pound in 1 day
c. 3 pounds in 1 week
d. 2 pounds in 1 day

46. According to the AHA/ACC/HRS guideline for the management of patients with atrial fibrillation, if a patient has atrial fibrillation or flutter that has lasted 48 hours or longer with duration known, how long should the patient receive treatment with warfarin prior to cardioversion?

a. No warfarin is recommended before cardioversion.
b. 2 weeks
c. 3 weeks
d. 4 weeks

47. The cardiac/vascular nurse has completed patient education about managing a patient's heart condition and wants to ensure that the patient has good retention. The best method to use is to:

a. Give a written quiz.
b. Utilize teach-back.
c. Ask if the patient has any questions.
d. Provide written instructions.

48. An older adult is to be discharged after having a heart attack but is at risk for impaired mobility and falls. When conducting a gait assessment as part of functional status, the cardiac/vascular nurse should be aware that the gait speed that is predictive of limitations is:

a. <0.6 meters/second
b. <0.8 meters/second
c. <1 meter/second
d. <1.5 meters/second

49. According to the AHA/AACVPR Core Components of Cardiac Rehabilitation, the 6-month minimum goal of weight loss for patients with BMI more than 25 and/or waist circumference more than 40 inches for males or more than 35 inches for females is:

a. ≥20%
b. ≥15%
c. ≥10%
d. ≥5%

50. Patients from which of the following ethnic/racial backgrounds are at the highest risk for cardiovascular disease?

a. Asian
b. Hispanic
c. African American
d. Caucasian

51. A widowed 70-year-old patient with vision impairment and rheumatoid arthritis lives alone and is being discharged from the hospital after an acute myocardial infarction and a prolonged stay. Which of the following is likely the most appropriate referral?

a. Telehealth service
b. Faith community nurse
c. Health navigator
d. Home health agency

52. The purpose of a health navigator is to help patients:

a. Through the continuum of care
b. Choose a health coverage option.
c. Choose an appropriate physician.
d. Understand different treatment options.

53. If the patient's telemetry shows a sinus rhythm with depressed ST segment and T-wave inversion, the cardiac/vascular nurse should suspect:

a. Myocardial ischemia
b. Myocardial injury
c. Myocardial infarction
d. Congenital abnormality

54. Under the Healthy People 2030 initiatives, the target mean total cholesterol level for people 20 years and older is:

a. 200 mg/dL
b. 197.7 mg/dL
c. 177.9 mg/dL
d. 186.4 mg/dL

55. For screening for cardiovascular risk in asymptomatic adults, which of the following is recommended or considered reasonable?

a. Genotype testing
b. Lipid parameters (lipoproteins, apolipoproteins, particle size, density)
c. Resting ECG
d. Echocardiogram

56. When utilizing the health belief model to help people to change behavior in order to manage chronic disease, the focus is on:

a. Negative consequences of current behavior
b. Positive outcomes from changes
c. Evaluating attitudes toward health
d. The power of emotions to bring about change

57. A patient has received an automatic implantable cardioverter-defibrillator (AICD) in the left chest. Instructions in the postoperative period should include to:

a. Call emergency medical services (EMS) for any shock, even if there are no ill effects.
b. Avoid lifting the left arm above the shoulder for four weeks.
c. Avoid walking for six weeks.
d. Avoid airports and building security systems.

58. The primary purpose of wearing a LifeVest is to:

a. Provide support of mid-sternal surgical incision.
b. Treat sudden cardiac arrest.
c. Monitor the heart rate and rhythm.
d. Monitor the effects of cardiac medications.

59. Which of the following is the strongest predictor of a person's health status?

a. Literacy skills
b. Age
c. Employment status
d. Income

60. If using the Modified Borg Scale for Perceived Dyspnea to evaluate endurance, severe shortness of breath is indicated by a score of:

a. 2
b. 5
c. 7
d. 10

61. When conducting the 6-minute walk test, which of the following is an indication that the test should be stopped immediately?

a. Patient exhibits moderate shortness of breath.
b. Patient complains of leg cramps.
c. Patient's face becomes flushed.
d. Patient begins to perspire slightly.

62. When administering the NIH stroke scale to a patient, the cardiac/vascular nurse should:

a. Conduct the test in the order items are listed.
b. Assess motor activity before cognitive activity.
c. Coach the patient through each section to optimize score.
d. Skip questions if the patient does not respond appropriately, and then redo them later.

63. The ankle-brachial index (ABI) of a patient is 0.85. This score indicates:

a. Severe peripheral arterial disease (PAD)
b. Calcified vessel (noncompressible)
c. Normal reading
d. Peripheral arterial disease (PAD)

64. The Pain Assessment in Advanced Dementia (PAINAD) scale evaluates 5 parameters: (1) respirations, (2) vocalization, (3) facial expression, (4) body language, and (5):

a. Combativeness
b. Responsiveness
c. Consolability
d. Cardiac rate

65. According to the ACC/AHA guidelines on the assessment of cardiac risk, the primary focus is on the lifetime risk for:

a. Myocardial infarction
b. Atherosclerotic cardiovascular disease (ASCVD)
c. Heart failure
d. Any type of cardiac disease

66. The Quality of Well-Being scale, Self-Administered (QWB-SA) assesses a period of:

a. 24 hours
b. 48 hours
c. 3 days
d. 6 days

67. Out of the 15 questions posed on the Short-Form Geriatric Depression Scale (GDS), what is the minimum number of "yes" answers that indicates the patient is experiencing depression?

a. 6
b. 7
c. 8
d. 10

68. Which of the following complementary therapies is likely to be the most effective for a patient with sinus tachycardia?

a. Acupuncture
b. Aromatherapy
c. Herbal medicine
d. Meditation

69. The apex of the heart can usually be auscultated at the left:

a. Third intercostal space
b. Fourth intercostal space
c. Fifth intercostal space
d. Sixth intercostal space

70. The first phase of the normal cardiac cycle is:

a. Ventricular ejection
b. Ventricular filling
c. Atrial systole
d. Isovolumetric ventricular contraction

71. The four key functions of cardiac cells are (1) automaticity, (2) excitability, (3) conductivity, and (4):

a. Contractility
b. Recovery
c. Repolarization
d. Transmission

72. According to the Society for Vascular Nursing clinical practice guideline for carotid artery stenting, which antiplatelet therapy is recommended pre-surgically?

a. Aspirin
b. Aspirin and clopidogrel
c. Ticlopidine
d. Prasugrel

73. When conducting a physical examination, the cardiac/vascular nurse finds the patient's blood pressure is elevated to 170/88 mmHg and pulse is 92 bpm. The nurse should:

a. Notify the physician immediately.
b. Take an ECG.
c. Repeat the BP and P in 5 minutes.
d. Complete the physical exam.

74. An S3 heart sound that occurs immediately after S2 over the mitral area is an indication of:

a. Systolic hypertension
b. Aortic stenosis
c. Left ventricular noncompliance
d. Right ventricular noncompliance

75. The normal range for a patient's pulse pressure is:

a. 10–20 mmHg
b. 30–50 mmHg
c. 50–70 mmHg
d. 70–80 mmHg

76. When assessing a patient's peripheral perfusion with the patient lying flat in supine position, before assisting the patient to sit up and dangle the legs, the nurse should:

a. Elevate one of the patient's legs 12 inches above the heart for 60 seconds.
b. Encourage the patient to take deep breaths and relax.
c. Elevate one of the patient's legs 6 inches off of the table for 60 seconds.
d. Ask the patient to flex and extend both feet for 30 seconds.

77. Capillary refill time of the finger nailbeds should not take more than:

a. 1 second
b. 2 seconds
c. 3 seconds
d. 4 seconds

78. When assessing for jugular venous distention, the patient should be positioned:

a. Flat and supine
b. Elevated to 45° and in lateral position
c. Elevated to 90° and supine
d. Elevated to 45° and supine

79. On physical examination, the cardiac/vascular nurse observes that the capillary refill time in the patient's finger is 7 seconds, and blanching of finger is followed by cyanosis and then erythema before normal color returns. These findings are consistent with:

a. Raynaud syndrome
b. Hypothermia
c. Cardiogenic shock
d. Acute arterial occlusion

80. A patient with jugular venous distention that is more pronounced on inspiration and who complains of chest pain and exhibits hepatosplenomegaly, ascites, and peripheral edema should be assessed for:

a. Muffled heart sounds
b. Pulsus paradoxus
c. Pericardial friction rub
d. Ventricular gallop

81. The cardiac enzyme or protein that is most specific to myocardial damage is:

a. Myoglobin
b. Troponin I
c. Troponin T
d. Creatine kinase-MB

82. The cardiac enzyme or protein that the cardiac/vascular nurse would expect to elevate first after an acute myocardial infarction is:

a. Myoglobin
b. Troponin I
c. Troponin T
d. Creatine kinase-MB

83. The PLAC and LDL tests are used to:

a. Predict the risk of heart failure.
b. Assess the degree of cardiac injury.
c. Predict the risk of coronary artery disease.
d. Evaluate response to statin therapy.

84. If a patient has impaired kidney function and is receiving low-molecular-weight heparin (LMWH), which of the following tests is most indicated to monitor heparin therapy?

a. INR
b. PT
c. aPTT
d. Anti-Xa

85. Following a cardiac arrest, which of the following treatments is best indicated to prevent neurological injury in unconscious survivors?

a. Intubation and ventilation
b. Therapeutic hypothermia
c. Frequent physical stimulation
d. Administration of steroids

86. If an outpatient was prescribed a beta-blocker for exertional angina and calls to report that he has seen no relief in 48 hours, the cardiac/vascular nurse should advise the patient to:

a. Expect the medication to take one to two weeks to begin to work.
b. Notify the physician immediately that the medication is not working.
c. Call 911 if the patient experiences any angina.
d. Avoid all exertion for at least four weeks.

87. Following a patient's myocardial infarction, the cardiac/vascular nurse needs to help the patient and family members understand (1) limitations, (2) improvement potential, and (3):

a. Precautions
b. Emotional changes
c. Complications
d. Support systems

88. The responsibility for being a change agent in an organization should fall on:

a. The administration
b. The nursing supervisors
c. Nurse educators
d. All personnel

89. In the role of preceptor for a graduate student, the cardiac/vascular nurse should expect the primary preceptor role to be to:

a. Supervise and guide the student.
b. Meet occasionally with the student.
c. Provide encouragement to the student.
d. Grade the student on achievement.

90. When the cardiac/vascular nurse is using the SBAR (situation-background-assessment-recommendation) method for the hand-off procedure at the end of shift, what information should the nurse convey as part of S (situation)?

a. Brief medical history
b. Patient's diagnosis
c. Plan for future procedures
d. Special needs

91. During presurgical preparations, the cardiac/vascular nurse notes that the patient seems well-informed and states she has no concerns but frequently rubs her hands together and tightly clasps her arms about her chest as well as sometimes staring at a picture on the wall. This nonverbal behavior suggests that the patient is:

a. Cold
b. Anxious
c. Bored
d. Disinterested

92. A patient with a poor prognosis is about to undergo emergent surgery for a dissecting aortic aneurysm and tells the cardiac/vascular nurse, "I'm probably not going to survive this operation." The best response is:

a. "It's a dangerous operation, but your surgeon is very skilled."
b. "I'm sorry, but you are right."
c. "What makes you feel that way?"
d. "Do you have any last wishes that you want me to convey?"

93. Which of the following drugs is commonly indicated for a patient with a hypertensive emergency and acute heart failure?

a. Esmolol hydrochloride
b. Nicardipine hydrochloride
c. Sodium nitroprusside
d. Labetalol hydrochloride

94. The most common complication after endovascular aneurysm repair (EVAR) of abdominal aortic aneurysm is:

a. Local wound infection
b. Access artery injury
c. Colonic ischemia
d. Endoleak

95. If the cardiac/vascular nurse finds in documenting in the electronic health record (EHR) that coded entries for some common signs and symptoms encountered in cardiac care are missing, the best solution is to:

a. Make free text entries.
b. Use the coded entries for similar problems.
c. Request information services add additional code.
d. Document on paper.

96. A 60-year-old patient who is to be discharged on a number of medications, including warfarin, must check his vital signs every day and have weekly blood tests. The patient states, "This is so much trouble! How can I keep track of everything?" The most therapeutic response is:

a. "Let's talk about this and work out a schedule together."
b. "Don't worry. It just seems confusing right now."
c. "You should try to make a simple schedule you can follow."
d. "You are right. There are a lot of things to keep track of."

97. Most medical assistance programs, such as those that provide drugs at low or no cost to patients, are available to patients based on:

a. Their diagnosis
b. Their age and disability
c. Their income
d. Physician referral

98. The cardiac/vascular nurse notes that a patient with a prosthetic heart valve has developed scattered petechiae on the body and splinter hemorrhages in the nail beds. Based on these observations, the cardiac/vascular nurse should suspect:

a. Coronary ischemia
b. Infectious endocarditis
c. Valve failure
d. Cardiomyopathy

99. An elderly Native American patient hospitalized with heart failure had been treated only by tribal healers until his illness became acute. The patient is very anxious in the hospital and suspicious and uncooperative with treatment. The best solution may be to:

a. Provide better education about the need for treatment.
b. Ask healers to participate in treatment.
c. Ask family members to intervene.
d. Ask tribal elders to direct the patient to be cooperative.

100. A patient who died in the cardiac care unit had confided to the cardiac/vascular nurse prior to her death that her daughter was not her husband's child and that she had never divulged this information but believed perhaps she should have. The nurse should:

a. Tell the husband.
b. Tell the daughter.
c. Maintain confidentiality.
d. Document the information in the patient's records.

101. A patient states that he has an advance directive and does not want to be resuscitated in the event of cardiac arrest or maintained on life support but is concerned his family may feel otherwise. The best advice the cardiac/vascular nurse can give the patient is to:

a. Not worry because his advance directive will be honored.
b. Discuss the matter with his family and let them know his wishes.
c. Tell the doctor about his wishes.
d. Make sure all health care providers have copies of the advance directive.

102. A patient who is recovering from insertion of a pacemaker because of bradycardia related to heart block tells the cardiac/vascular nurse that she worries about living with cardiac disease and needs more information. The best referral is probably to the:

a. Mended Hearts
b. American Heart Association
c. Patient's physician
d. Internet

103. An older patient became very confused, climbed out of bed, and slipped on the floor, fracturing a hip. The patient's family is meeting with personnel from risk management. The primary purpose of risk management is to:

a. Settle issues out of court.
b. Assess the degree of a problem.
c. Offer solutions to problems that arise.
d. Anticipate problems and resolve them.

104. A patient in the cardiac care unit is nonresponsive and on life support, and his two daughters are in complete disagreement about his treatment. If the cardiac/vascular nurse comes into the room and finds them loudly arguing, the best response is:

a. "You need to take this argument elsewhere."
b. "How would your father feel about your arguing?"
c. "Let's sit down together and talk about this."
d. "You really need to make a decision about your father."

105. The wife of a patient who has experienced a severe myocardial infarction and is doing poorly has started spending hours in the hospital chapel praying and states that she believes God will save her husband. According to Kübler-Ross's five stages of grief, the stage of grief that the wife is probably undergoing is:

a. Denial
b. Bargaining
c. Depression
d. Acceptance

106. When monitoring a patient's telemetry, the cardiac/vascular nurse notes that the mean arterial pressure (MAP) has dropped from 70 to 55 mmHg. The nurse's immediate response should be to:

a. Administer oxygen and notify the MD.
b. Raise patient's head to 45 degrees.
c. Change the patient's position.
d. Administer nitroglycerine.

107. If a patient who is a Jehovah's Witness is to undergo emergent angiography and angioplasty, the most important religion-related question to ask the patient is if she:

a. Wants a minister called
b. Will accept blood products
c. Will take medications
d. Wants a faith healer called

108. The approach most commonly used for transcatheter aortic valve replacement (TAVR) is:

a. Transfemoral
b. Transaortic
c. Transapical
d. Transradial

109. The physician has reviewed the consent forms with a patient and the patient has signed prior to surgery, but the patient appears to believe he is having a noninvasive procedure rather than the open-heart procedure scheduled. The nurse should:

a. Tell the patient that he is wrong.
b. Report the physician to administration.
c. Call the physician and report the patient's misconception.
d. Notify surgery to cancel the procedure.

110. If a patient qualifies for home health care under Medicare (Original), Medicare will pay the agency a fee based on the patient's condition for an "episode of care," which is a period of:

a. 30 days
b. 60 days
c. 90 days
d. 120 days

111. The purpose of Home and Community-Based Services (HCBS) programs provided through Medicaid is to:

a. Maintain patients in their home environments rather than nursing homes.
b. Reduce the overall cost of caring for patients.
c. Place patients into appropriate nursing homes for care.
d. Provide home health care for patients recently hospitalized.

112. The cardiac/vascular nurse needs to delegate personal care of a stable but anxious patient who has recently undergone open-heart surgery and still has drains and IVs in place. The available personnel include a newly graduated LVN with no experience in the unit, a CNA who has worked in the unit for 5 years, and a CNA who has worked in the unit for 6 weeks. By delegating this task to the CNA who has worked on the unit for 5 years over the new LVN with more extensive education, the nurse is demonstrating which "right" of delegation?

a. Right circumstance
b. Right task
c. Right person
d. Right supervision and evaluation

113. If the cardiac/vascular nurse believes that a procedure can be effectively shortened without any compromise in quality, the next step should be to:

a. Ask other staff if they agree.
b. Suggest the supervisor give the procedure a trial period.
c. Shorten the procedure when utilizing it.
d. Write a formal proposal for change.

114. The type of coping strategy that a patient is exhibiting when the patient constantly asks questions and utilizes Internet searches to obtain information about all treatments and medications is:

a. Being optimistic
b. Using social support
c. Accepting the situation
d. Trying to maintain control

115. When users of the new electronic health record (EHR) were evaluated, the cardiac/vascular nurse was the only nurse on the unit with no errors in documentation, while many others were struggling to utilize the new system correctly. Because of this, the cardiac/vascular nurse should:

a. Suggest the other nurses ask for more training.
b. Offer to serve as a resource person.
c. Ask for a raise in pay.
d. Advise the other nurses they need to be more careful.

116. Following a carotid endarterectomy, a patient exhibits bradycardia, weak tone of voice, and dysphagia. The most likely reason is trauma to the:

a. Vagus nerve (X) (superior laryngeal)
b. Glossopharyngeal nerve (IX)
c. Spinal accessory nerve (XI)
d. Hypoglossal nerve (XII)

117. When assessing cardiovascular function, the two most important symptoms to question the patient about are:

a. Pain and edema
b. Pain and shortness of breath
c. Weight gain and pain
d. Pain and palpitations

118. Which of the following tasks can be delegated to unlicensed assistive personnel?

a. Determining interventions needed in the plan of care
b. Checking a patient's vital signs during an episode of chest pain
c. Identifying goals related to the nursing diagnosis
d. Emptying a urinary catheter bag and measuring the urine

119. Which type of defense mechanism is a patient utilizing when the patient refuses to get out of bed or attend to any self-care and leaves decision-making to the patient's spouse?

a. Dissociation
b. Denial
c. Regression
d. Assertiveness

120. If the cardiac/vascular nurse is caring for a close friend of a nurse on another unit and the nurse asks about the results of the patient's laboratory tests, the best response is:

a. "I'm sorry, I can't give you that information."
b. "You should know that's a HIPAA violation."
c. "They were within normal range, so don't worry."
d. "I'll get you a copy of the results."

121. According to the Eighth Report of the Joint National Committee on Prevention, Detection, Evaluation, and Treatment of High Blood Pressure, a 62-year-old patient should be treated for hypertension with medications if their blood pressure is:

a. 120/90 mmHg or higher
b. 130/90 mmHg or higher
c. 140/90 mmHg or higher
d. 150/90 mmHg or higher

122. A patient's nursing diagnoses include (1) risk for fluid volume excess related to heart failure, (2) risk for ineffective coping related to change in status, (3) imbalanced nutrition, more than body requirements related to poor food choices and knowledge deficit, and (4) acute pain related to myocardial infarction. The diagnoses should be prioritized (first to last) for interventions in the following order:

a. Acute pain, risk for fluid volume excess, imbalanced nutrition, and ineffective coping
b. Risk for fluid volume excess, ineffective coping, imbalanced nutrition, and acute pain
c. Risk for fluid volume excess, acute pain, imbalanced nutrition, and ineffective coping
d. Acute pain, risk for fluid volume excess, ineffective coping, and imbalanced nutrition

123. A patient with chronic heart failure and reduced cardiac output has an ejection fraction (EF) of 33%. An appropriate expected outcome of treatment is:

a. EF ≥35%
b. EF ≥40%
c. EF ≥60%
d. EF ≥65%

124. If a patient has been prescribed simvastatin or atorvastatin for high cholesterol, which of the following foods/drinks should be limited?

a. Cranberry juice
b. Black licorice
c. Milk
d. Grapefruit juice

125. Patients taking loop and/or thiazide diuretics should be routinely monitored for:

a. Calcium levels
b. Vitamin D levels
c. Potassium levels
d. Sodium levels

126. Which of the follow comorbidities precludes the use of a beta-blocker for treatment of heart disease?

a. Severe asthma
b. Cancer
c. Rheumatoid arthritis
d. Osteoporosis

127. A patient receiving digoxin 0.25 mg daily had a recent digoxin level of 1.8 ng/mL (normal therapeutic levels are 0.5–2.0 ng/mL) but is exhibiting a pulse rate of 56 bpm with occasional dysrhythmia. The cardiac/vascular nurse should:

a. Administer the digoxin.
b. Withhold the digoxin.
c. Withhold the digoxin and begin ECG monitoring.
d. Administer the digoxin and begin ECG monitoring.

128. The Unna boot is contraindicated for patients who have:

a. Pitting edema
b. Venous ulcers
c. Venous insufficiency
d. Nonambulatory status

129. The primary reason for beginning cardiac rehabilitation while the patient is still in the acute hospital is to:

a. Begin adaptive training.
b. Prevent negative results of deconditioning.
c. Prepare the patient psychologically for recovery.
d. Prevent further cardiac events.

130. In an older adult, key indications of coronary artery disease are:

a. Chest and neck pain
b. Chest pain and nausea
c. Epigastric discomfort and fatigue
d. Fatigue and dyspnea

131. A patient with hypertrophic cardiomyopathy is especially at risk for:

a. Ascites
b. Anemia
c. Sudden cardiac death
d. Hepatosplenomegaly

132. The ECG changes that are common to myocardial injury and myocardial infarction include:

a. ST-segment elevation and T-wave inversion
b. ST-segment depression and T-wave inversion
c. Prolonged QT segment with T-wave inversion
d. T-wave inversion and absent P wave

133. Which of the following is an absolute contraindication to thrombolytic use for a myocardial infarction?

a. Current anticoagulation therapy with warfarin (INR at least 2–3)
b. Internal bleeding within 2–4 weeks
c. Suspected aortic dissection
d. History of chronic, severe, poorly controlled hypertension

134. When reviewing a patient's list of medications, the cardiac/vascular nurse notes that, in addition to apixaban, the patient takes paroxetine, levothyroxine, dioctyl sodium sulfosuccinate (DSS or docusate sodium), and hydrochlorothiazide. Which of these drugs may interact with apixaban to increase the risk of bleeding?

a. Paroxetine
b. Levothyroxine
c. DSS
d. Hydrochlorothiazide

135. According to the AHA/ACC/HRS guideline for the management of patients with atrial fibrillation, the recommended antithrombotic therapy for patients with mechanical heart valves and atrial fibrillation is:

a. Unfractionated heparin
b. Warfarin
c. Aspirin
d. Rivaroxaban

136. If the corrected QT (cQT) interval is 0.42 seconds at a standardized heart rate of 60 bpm, approximately what is the estimated expected cQT for a patient with a heart rate of 90 bpm?

a. 0.48 seconds
b. 0.46 seconds
c. 0.38 seconds
d. 0.36 seconds

137. When using a radial pressure device to promote hemostasis after an arterial blood draw, once the pressure device is applied, it should be left in place initially for:

a. 5 minutes
b. 10 minutes
c. 20 minutes
d. 30 minutes

138. If a patient must have an IV inserted and blood tests but states that she is terrified of needles and may faint, the best course of action is to:

a. Ask the patient what might help relieve her anxiety.
b. Suggest the physician order an antianxiety medication.
c. Advise the patient to take deep breaths and try to relax.
d. Reassure the patient that the procedures will not be painful.

139. According to the AHA/ACC/HRS guideline for the management of patients with atrial fibrillation, in order to successfully maintain sinus rhythm after cardioversion for atrial fibrillation, the atrial fibrillation should have had a duration of:

a. <1 month
b. <3 months
c. <6 months
d. <12 months

140. When a patient is undergoing cardiac rehabilitation, a measure that may be used for the behavioral outcome domain is:

a. Percent of body fat
b. Exercise regimen
c. Mortality
d. Patient satisfaction

141. First-degree relatives of patients with familial dilated cardiomyopathy should be screened for the disorders with:

a. ECGs every year
b. CTA and physical exam every year
c. Serial echocardiography every 3–5 years
d. Serial echocardiography every year

142. When assessing the cardiovascular system of an older adult, the cardiac/vascular nurse should expect:

a. Posterior displacement of the apical pulse
b. Narrowed pulse pressure
c. Amplified heart sounds
d. Decreased systolic blood pressure

143. When assessing a patient, the cardiac/vascular nurse notes central cyanosis. What does this likely indicate?

a. Reduction in blood flow
b. Reduction in body temperature
c. Reduction in RBC count
d. Reduction in oxygen saturation

144. If a patient is having a pharmacologic echocardiogram with IV dipyridamole and develops shortness of breath and dizziness, which of the following medications should the cardiac/vascular nurse expect to administer to relieve the adverse effects?

a. Dobutamine
b. Aminophylline
c. Compazine
d. Corticosteroid

145. How many calories per day is the DASH eating plan to control hypertension based on?

a. 1000 calories
b. 1400 calories
c. 1600 calories
d. 2000 calories

146. A patient is prescribed metoprolol for control of supraventricular tachycardia and hypertension. The cardiac/vascular nurse should advise the patient to:

a. Take the mediation with food.
b. Take the medication in the evening.
c. Avoid abruptly stopping the medication.
d. Avoid taking the medication with milk.

147. For health promotion, a primary prevention of hypertension includes:

a. A public campaign to promote exercise
b. Screening patients for high blood pressure
c. Cardiac rehabilitation program
d. Support group for patients with cardiovascular disease

148. If a patient shows nonverbal indications of pain (tense, withdrawn, frowning, holding her chest) as well as increased respiratory and heart rate but describes pain on a 1-to-10 scale as "2," the cardiac/vascular nurse should:

a. Assume the patient is not in acute pain.
b. Ask the patient about pain in another way.
c. Assume the patient is stoic and simply denying pain.
d. Explain the 1-to-10 scale again.

149. A 70-year-old man is undergoing cardiac rehabilitation after a severe myocardial infarction but is very anxious about the change in his physical condition and lacks family and social support. The most applicable nursing diagnosis is:

a. Risk of ineffective coping
b. Ineffective protection
c. Deficient knowledge
d. Risk for spiritual distress

150. If a fellow nurse for whom the cardiac/vascular nurse is serving as a mentor gave a patient the wrong dose of a medication, the best response for the mentor is:

a. "You are lucky you didn't get fired!"
b. "I hope you learned how important double-checking is."
c. "What did you learn from this experience?"
d. "You poor thing! You must be so upset."

Answer Key and Explanations for Test #1

1. B: Atrial fibrillation is defined in terms of duration and response to treatment. Definitions of atrial fibrillation include:

- Paroxysmal: ends spontaneously or with treatment within 1 week
- Persistent: continues for more than 1 week
- Longstanding: continues for more than 1 year
- Permanent: has not responded to treatment, and patient and clinician agree to stop further attempts—at least for the present—to convert the fibrillation to sinus rhythm

2. D: The PQRST method of angina assessment includes:

- (P) Precipitating factors: events that preceded the episode of pain, such as exercise, eating, or arguing
- (Q) Quality of pain: dull, aching, sharp, tight, heavy, or squeezing
- (R) Radiation of pain: location of pain and radiation to outside of the chest (neck, arms, back, jaw, or shoulder)
- (S) Severity of pain
- (T) Timing: onset of pain, persistence, first-time pain, or recurrent

3. A: When teaching a patient with coronary artery disease to control angina, the first step is to determine what precipitates episodes because patients may not have made a correlation between activity and pain, and in some cases, patients need to modify their work or lifestyle in order to prevent angina from occurring. Other important things to discuss include coping mechanisms, taking medications correctly, maintaining a healthy diet, and engaging in regular exercises to tolerance (under the guidance of a physician).

4. C: Using a bedside commode is a moderate-energy activity (3–6 METs). Activity classifications include:

- Low energy (<3 METs): simple activities such as eating and washing the face and hands or resting
- Moderate energy (3–6 METs): using a bedside commode, taking a shower, walking at 3–4 miles per hour, and using a bedpan
- High energy (6–8 METs): walking 5 miles per hour and ascending a flight of stairs
- Very high energy (≥9 METs): running or other strenuous physical activity

5. D: If PCI, such as coronary angioplasty, is to be used to treat a patient with an acute MI with occluded coronary artery, the PCI should be performed within 90 minutes. If PCI is carried out within a short period of time after the cardiac event by experienced clinicians, the results are comparable with results achieved with thrombolysis. Complications can include subacute occlusion of stents, restenosis (usually late-occurring), hematoma formation at catheter insertion site, arterial thrombosis, and local and/or systemic infection.

6. B: If telemetry shows a regular heart rate of 64 bpm with normal P wave, normal QRS complex, and PR interval of 0.25 seconds, the heart rhythm would be classified as exhibiting first-degree AV block because of the prolonged PR interval (>0.2 seconds). With first-degree AV block, all impulses are transmitted to the ventricles, but the duration of the conduction is longer than normal. No treatment other than monitoring or adjusting causative agents (such as medications) is indicated.

7. A: Because the patient's symptoms (pain and tenderness in the right posterior thigh) are consistent with deep vein thrombosis (DVT) (probably provoked by hospitalization), the patient should immediately be placed on bedrest and the leg elevated until radiologic diagnostic tests are completed. Treatment usually includes warm, moist compresses as well as rest and elevation, but the primary treatment is anticoagulation, especially for proximal DVT of the upper leg because proximal DVTs carry higher mortality rates than distal.

8. C: As part of the US Department of Health and Human Services' 5 A's (ask, advise, assess, assist, and arrange follow-up) guidelines for smoking cessation, during the "assist" stage, patients should be asked to establish a target date for quitting that is within 14 days because if the target date is further away, the patient is less likely to follow through. The cardiac/vascular nurse should assist the patient to make a plan for quitting that includes removing all cigarettes and asking family and friends to assist. The need for abstinence rather than trying to slowly withdraw cigarettes should be stressed.

9. C: The intensity of a heart murmur that is loud and accompanied by a thrill would be classified as grade III/VI. Grades range from I to VI (always expressed in Roman numerals) and notation is written as "(finding)/VI." Grades include:

I. Barely detectible
II. Soft and quiet
III. Loud with a thrill
IV. Very loud with thrust or thrill
V. Extremely loud and detectible before the stethoscope makes contact with the skin

10. B: According to the National Heart, Lung, and Blood Institute Adult Treatment Panel III (ATP III) recommendations for cholesterol management, the primary target of therapy for LDL (low-density lipoprotein) cholesterol is below 100 mg/dL. LDL classification is as follows:

<100	Optimal
100–129	Near optimal/above optimal
130–159	Borderline high
160–189	High
≥190	Very high

Total cholesterol should be maintained below 200 mg/dL. HDL (high-density lipoprotein) is low if it is below 40 mg/dL and high if it is ≥60 mg/dL. High risk factors for coronary heart disease events include coronary heart disease, symptomatic carotid artery disease, peripheral arterial disease, and abdominal aortic aneurysm.

11. C: B-type natriuretic peptide (BNP) is the best marker for ventricular dysfunction and heart failure. BNP is a hormone secreted by the ventricular tissues in response to increased pressure in the ventricles and increased volume, such as may occur with heart failure. BNP promotes vasodilation and sodium excretion and may attenuate sympathetic activation, which stimulates the release of catecholamines and results in vasoconstriction. Normal values are <100 pg/mL; levels of 100–300 pg/mL indicate beginning heart failure. The level for mild heart failure is >300 pg/mL; the level for moderate heart failure is >600 pg/mL; and the level for severe heart failure is >900 pg/mL.

12. A: When using the SMART format to develop targeted goals, these goals should be:

- (S) Specific: should clearly outline what is to be accomplished, by whom, and the timeline
- (M) Measurable: should include concrete measurements that help the patient to stay focused on the goal and to observe progress
- (A) Attainable: should be reasonable and within the capacity of the patient
- (R) Realistic: should represent a goal that the patient is willing to work toward
- (T) Timely: should include a firm time frame so that the patient can measure achievement against time

13. B: When a patient is faced with a serious illness, the most effective initial intervention to assist the patient with coping skills is to use a calm and reassuring approach, as this can help the patient to stay focused and to avoid panic. When the patient is receptive, the nurse can ask about past coping skills and discuss techniques for coping, such as relaxation exercises. Providing factual information about the disease can often help allay concerns.

14. A: If a unit supervisor is considering a switch in policy that affects staff members and a meeting is called to discuss the issues, the first step in resolving the conflict should be to allow both sides to present their opinions about the issue, keeping the focus on the issue rather than individuals. The discussion should generate pro and con lists so that each side of the conflict has a clear understanding of the issues involved to determine if a consensus can be reached.

15. D: The troponin I level that indicates cardiac injury is >0.04 ng/mL. The normal level is 0.0–0.04 ng/mL (may vary according to reference lab). Troponin I levels increase about 3-6 hours after damage to the myocardium and peak in 14–20 hours, returning to the baseline rate within about 7–10 days. Troponin T, which is less specific, remains elevated for longer periods, up to about 2 weeks, so the troponins are preferred for early detection of MI as well as late detection.

16. C: According to the American College of Cardiology Foundation (ACCF)/American Heart Association (AHA) heart failure guideline, the most important intervention for the treatment of stage A heart failure is controlling hypertension, with long-term treatment of both systolic and diastolic hypertension cutting the risk of heart failure in half. First-line treatment is diuretics, which are well tolerated by most patients. Other acceptable treatments, depending on the patient's condition, include beta-blockers, ACE inhibitors, and ARBs. Treatment of dyslipidemia is also considered of primary importance. Other recommendations include reduction in obesity and control of hyperglycemia in diabetic patients.

17. D: In the design of the delivery system under the Chronic Care Model of disease management, patients should be provided care that is understandable and culturally appropriate. The Chronic Care Model is proactive in that the goal is to prevent complications and maintain the patient in optimum health. Patient needs should be identified, and interventions should be evidence-based. Patients should receive case management and regular follow-up by team members who have defined roles.

18. B: When utilizing the $CHADS_2$ stratification score to estimate stroke risk for patients with nonvalvular atrial fibrillation, each increase of 1 point in the scale increases risk of stroke by approximately 2 percent, although this estimate holds better for patients on the lower end of the scale than the upper, as the risk increases more at scores of 5 and 6. The $CHADS_2$ score assigns points for conditions that increase risk, with scores ranging from 0 (1.9% risk) to 6 (18.2%):

- Congestive heart failure: 1
- Hypertension: 1
- Age ≥75: 1
- Stroke/transient ischemic attack (TIA)/thromboembolism (TE): 2

19. A: Pitting edema (moderate to severe) is associated with peripheral venous insufficiency. Other indications of peripheral venous insufficiency include irregular-shaped ulcerations of the medial or lateral malleolus and the anterior tibial area. Pedal pulses are present but may be difficult to palpate if the edema is severe, and the patient may complain of aching and cramping of the legs. Brownish discoloration (hemosiderosis) is often evident around the ankles and anterior tibial areas. Patients may exhibit varicosities.

20. B: If a patient is brought to the ED after collapsing at a public event and is believed to have had a myocardial infarction, but the patient adamantly refuses all care because she is a Christian Scientist, the best response of the nurse is, "Let's talk about lifestyle changes that may help." Patients have the right to refuse any and all treatments even though that refusal may lead to their deaths, and religious beliefs can be very strong, so the cardiac/vascular nurse should focus on what the patient may agree to, such as smoking cessation, limiting activity, and diet modification.

21. A: The key component of health promotion is personal responsibility because the individual is ultimately responsible for making the necessary lifestyle changes. Encouraging people to take responsibility may include educational programs, although education alone is often not adequate to change behavior, especially if patients lack motivation. Some patients may respond to a rewards program or to the personal rewards that come from making changes. Research shows that no one type of program works better than any other because of individual factors.

22. C: If a patient repeatedly asks, "Can I take notes?" during a demonstration of a dressing change procedure, the patient's preferred learning style is probably read-write. VARK classification includes:

- Visual: prefers visual illustrations, such as pictures, videos, and flowcharts, which outline directions step by step
- Aural: prefers to listen to directions and to discuss the steps to a procedure
- Read-write: prefers to learn by reading and may rely on extensive note-taking during instructions in order to stay focused on the material
- Kinesthetic: prefers hands-on techniques that allow the person to manipulate supplies and carry out the steps to a procedure with minimal instruction

23. B: In the ARCS model of motivational design (Keller), the aspect that focuses on the learner's experience is relevance:

- Attention: focuses on methods to gain attention, such as encouraging active participation, giving variable presentations, introducing opposing positions/controversies, utilizing humor, and providing specific examples
- Relevance: focuses on ways the learner can use the material by connecting it to previous experience, presenting the value and usefulness, matching it to the learner's needs, and modeling (guest speakers, videos)

- Confidence: focuses on assisting the learner to believe in successful learning by providing objective and learning criteria, providing feedback, and promoting autonomy
- Satisfaction: focuses on the rewards of learning without being patronizing

24. A: When conducting a motivational interview, the initial assessment should be related to cognitive variables, which include the patient's capacity to learn (intellectual ability) and mental readiness (desire, curiosity). Other variables include affective variables (level of anxiety, emotional state), physiological variables (physical abilities and/or limitations), experiential variables (previous experiences), environmental variables (setting, family/social support), and the relationship between the patient and the nurse (positive or negative). Subjective measurement of a patient's motivation depends on self-report and observation. Objective measurement is indirect and relates to quantifying observations.

25. C: Food diaries are commonly used to assess patient's diets. The Fat-Related Diet Habits Questionnaire asks questions about food intake over the previous 1-month period, but recall is often impaired, so a food diary is a valuable addition. The food diary should include at least 1 leisure (not at work) day because food consumption may change depending on work status. Studies have shown that the reliability of reporting decreases after 3 days because the act of reporting may alter eating habits.

26. B: When planning an educational program about lifestyle changes for a cardiac rehabilitation program, the cardiac/vascular nurse recognizes that most adult learners are self-directed. Because they are used to being autonomous, the nurse should allow adult learners as much autonomy as possible, emphasizing their control over the learning process. Adults also often prefer a problem-oriented approach as opposed to a subject-oriented approach. Adults may have experiential learning that allows them to reason at an advanced level.

27. D: When assessing a patient's readiness to learn, an example of experiential learning is a previous coping mechanism. Readiness factors include:

- Physical: gender, health status, physical abilities/disabilities, effects of the environment, and the skills needed for the complexity of the task
- Emotional: the patient's anxiety level, support system, motivation, attitude, developmental stage, and evidence of risk-taking behavior (drinking, drug use, gambling, extreme sports)
- Experiential: includes not only past coping mechanisms but the patient's experiences based on cultural background and orientation and the patient's degree of control
- Knowledge: cognitive ability, learning style, knowledge base, and learning disabilities (such as dyslexia)

28. D: If a patient with suspected hypertensive crisis presents with BP 200/125 mmHg, the patient's mean arterial pressure (MAP) is 150 mmHg. The formula for MAP is:

$$\text{MAP} = \frac{\text{Diastole} \times 2 + \text{Systole}}{3} = \frac{125 \times 2 + 200}{3} = \frac{450}{3} = 150$$

During treatment for hypertensive crisis, the MAP is often used instead of the BP to guide therapy, with the initial goal to decrease MAP by no more than 25% within minutes to an hour because too rapid decrease in BP can result in decreased cerebral, renal, and coronary perfusion, and could cause a stroke.

29. C: Red yeast rice is a complementary/alternative therapy that scientific studies show may decrease LDL, triglycerides, and total cholesterol, as it is a natural statin (although in lower doses than prescribed medications, and dosages are not standardized, so effects may vary). Garlic, despite anecdotal reports, does not affect cholesterol levels. Omega-3 fatty acids may reduce triglyceride levels. Plant sterols may reduce total cholesterol.

30. A: When a patient has an implantable cardioverter-defibrillator, overdrive pacing is utilized for ventricular tachycardia. ICDs monitor heart rate and rhythm. About 25 seconds after a lethal dysrhythmia is detected, the ICD delivers a shock to the patient's heart and then a second shock if the first is not successful. Additionally, the ICD contains pacemakers for bradycardia and tachycardia, so when supraventricular or ventricular tachycardias occur, the overdrive pacing takes over to prevent the need for the shock.

31. C: When charged with educating patients about self-care after they have undergone outpatient cardiac procedures, the factor that is most likely to be a barrier to learning is time constraints. Patients often arrive shortly before the scheduled procedure, and there is little time for education during preparation. Following the procedure, when the patient has recovered enough to be receptive to learning, the patient is usually preparing for discharge, so discharge instructions are too often reviewed very quickly or simply given to the patient in written form. For this reason, follow-up after discharge is important.

32. B: When a patient with dilated cardiomyopathy (or any type of cardiomyopathy) is to be discharged, family members should be advised to take a CPR course because cardiomyopathy places the patient at increased risk of sudden cardiac death. The family should also be advised when to call 911. Dilated cardiomyopathy is the result of damage to muscle fibers of the heart, interfering with myocardial metabolism and resulting in dilation of all heart chambers. Prognosis is poor because the condition is usually advanced before symptoms are evident.

33. D: An example of a well-written measurable objective is: "Following one-on-one instruction about weight loss, the patient will be able to list four strategies for weight loss." The four-part method is often used to write effective specific objectives, which are not only prescriptive but also measurable:

1. Condition/testing circumstance: "Following one-on-one instruction about weight loss"
2. Learner: "the patient"
3. Performance: "will be able to list"
4. Criterion: "Four strategies for weight loss."

34. A: While all of these needs are important, the primary concern for discharge planning should be care and service needs. Patients are usually discharged on statins and beta-blockers, and, if exhibiting prolonged abnormal heart rhythm after coming off of bypass, warfarin. Patients need to be educated about the medications, including possible adverse reactions. They may need to monitor their heart rate and blood pressure, weight, exercise, and diet, and these multiple demands may be overwhelming to patients. Some patients may require home health care after discharge until their conditions are more stable.

35. B: For a 62-year-old man with supraventricular tachycardia (SVT) exhibiting a normal pulse rate on metoprolol but elevated blood pressure, the risk factor that most needs modification is the patient's smoking 1 pack of cigarettes daily because smoking poses the greatest potential for harm. The patient should limit wine to 1–2 glasses daily and should increase exercise to 150 minutes per week. While patients with SVT are usually advised to avoid caffeine, tea has lower levels of caffeine than coffee, but the patient should switch to decaffeinated tea.

36. D: According to the American Heart Association guidelines for exercise, the target heart rate for a patient who is 65 years old and engaging in moderate exercises is 78–132 bpm, depending on the patient's pulse at rest (average is 60–100 bpm for older adults). The average maximum heart rate for a patient this age is 155 bpm, and the target should be to attain 50–85% of that rate during exercise. (Using the formula of 220 minus the person's age provides an estimation of maximum heart rate for age.)

37. D: If a patient with paroxysmal SVT is to have mobile cardiac event monitoring for a 1-month period with 3 leads connected to a transmitter that sends a message to a cellphone that transmits ECGs to the company, the maximum distance that the patient should be from the cellphone is 10 feet. The patient should attach both the transmitter and the cellphone to her waist or carry the phone in a pocket or purse.

38. C: While clarity, timeliness, and knowledge are all important, the most important factor in interdisciplinary communication is respect and the ability to demonstrate appreciation for the contributions of others. All health care providers involved in a patient's care have important yet different roles. When problems arise, it is not uncommon for one department to lay blame on another department, but this approach is nonproductive, as it can result in impaired communication and further problems.

39. D: If the cardiac/vascular nurse is interested in advocating for the advancement of nursing practice, the most effective method is to become involved in national organizations, such as the American Nurses Association (ANA) and Preventive Cardiovascular Nurses Association (PCNA), as these organizations are often active in lobbying political bodies and developing guidelines for health care. Organizations often have many committees on which a nurse can serve. The cardiac/vascular nurse can also make presentations at conferences at the local, state, and national levels.

40. A: If a 58-year-old female patient whose blood pressure had been well controlled during acute and convalescent hospitalization has shown increasing blood pressure readings for the past few weeks since discharge and gives vague responses about the medication, the cardiac/vascular nurse should first address nonadherence. After several weeks, the patient should know what medications she is taking, but her statement ("I have the directions written down at home") suggests that she does not and may need more education and supervision.

41. C: If a patient cannot be weaned off of cardiopulmonary bypass (CPB) after severe acute myocardial injury, the intervention most indicated is a left ventricular assist device (LVAD). If the patient stays on CPB for prolonged periods, the patient may develop severe coagulopathy, so the decision to transition to LVAD must be made quickly. The LVAD decreases the work of the LV and maintains systolic blood pressure while giving the LV time to heal, but recovery should begin within 30 hours or risk of death is high.

42. B: In traditional Islamic culture, such as that of Saudi Arabia, the man makes decisions, so a woman would defer decisions to her husband; however, when it comes to personal care, such as attending to a wound or changing dressings, these tasks would be the responsibility of a woman. In this case, the patient's mother would likely be responsible for providing wound care unless she is unable to do so, and then the duty would fall to the adolescent daughter.

43. C: If a patient has an electrically-powered LVAD with a portable battery pack to use when moving about and wants to increase activity level, the patient should increase the pump speed to compensate for the increased activity, but the patient should receive instruction about adjusting the pump speed and should practice under supervised conditions before discharge, and the patient should be apprised of limitations to activities to prevent increased demand on the heart.

44. A: A patient who has minimal chest pain on exertion but none at rest and whose coronary angiography shows 90% blockage of the left main coronary artery would be classified according to the NYHA functional classification for heart failure as functional capacity 2, objective assessment D. Functional capacity is categorized as class (1) no problem with activity, (2) minimal symptoms with activity, (3) markedly limited physical ability, and (4) symptoms at rest. Objective assessment includes (A) no evidence of disease, (B) evidence of minimal disease, (C) evidence of moderately severe disease, and (D) evidence of severe disease.

45. D: The weight gains that may indicate heart failure are 1–3 pounds in 1 day or 5 pounds in 1 week. Patients with heart failure should keep daily weights, usually each morning at the same time, and should notify the clinician if weight gain suggests heart failure because sudden weight gain may be life-threatening, especially if pulmonary edema develops. Patients may develop peripheral edema, decreased frequency of urination, dyspnea, and cough as well as increased weakness.

46. C: According to the AHA/ACC/HRS guideline for the management of patients with atrial fibrillation, if a patient has atrial fibrillation or flutter that has lasted 48 hours or longer with duration known, the patient should receive treatment with warfarin for at least 3 weeks prior to cardioversion (target INR of 2–3) and should continue on warfarin for 4 weeks after cardioversion to reduce the risk of heart attack or stroke resulting from an embolism.

47. B: The best method to use to ensure that a patient has good retention after completing patient education is to utilize the teach-back method. For this method, the nurse goes through the information slowly, and upon completion asks a question to prompt the patient to teach back the information: "How would you explain what you need to do to your family?" This allows the nurse to assess the patient's retention and understanding and to identify areas that need reinforcement.

48. A: When conducting a gait assessment as part of functional status, the cardiac/vascular nurse should be aware that the gait speed that is predictive of limitations is less than 0.6 meters/second. For the test, the patient should be observed while walking for 5 meters in a previously measured area, and a stopwatch should be used to note the time. Functional assessment may also include the timed up and go (TUG) test and performance-oriented mobility assessment (POMA).

49. D: According to the AHA/AACVPR Core Components of Cardiac Rehabilitation, the 6-month minimal goal of weight loss for patients with BMI more than 25 and/or waist circumference more than 40 inches for males or more than 35 inches for females is at least 5%, although more than 10% is the optimal goal. Weight loss should result from a combination of diet, exercise, and behavioral modifications. Expected short-term outcome is that the patient's progress will be evaluated, and program modifications will be made as needed. The expected long-term outcome is continued adherence to the program.

50. C: African American patients are at the highest risk for cardiovascular disease, with rates of heart failure occurring before age 50 that are 20 times higher than for Caucasians. Even young children show increased cholesterol levels and excessive weight. Cardiovascular disease is the leading cause of death among both male and female African Americans, and statistics show that the rates of cardiovascular disease among African Americans who are age 20 and older range from 44% (male) to 49% (female).

51. D: The most appropriate referral for a widowed 70-year-old patient with vision impairment and rheumatoid arthritis who lives alone and is being discharged from the hospital after an acute myocardial infarction and a prolonged stay is likely the home health agency. The home health agency can provide nursing services to monitor the patient's condition and a home health aide to assist with personal care. Because the patient's condition should render the patient essentially homebound, the patient qualifies for coverage under Medicare.

52. B: The purpose of a health navigator is to help patients choose a health coverage option from the health insurance marketplace. A health navigator may be an individual or an organization, but the navigator must be trained in assisting individuals and must be able to help them complete eligibility and enrollment forms. There is no charge for the health navigator service, which is provided as part of the Affordable Care Act.

53. A: If the patient's telemetry shows a sinus rhythm with depressed ST segment and T-wave inversion, the cardiac/vascular nurse should suspect myocardial ischemia resulting from impaired coronary artery circulation. If the ST segment becomes elevated, then this indicates myocardial damage and possible myocardial infarction. With ischemia, the patient may complain of angina or pain in the neck, jaw, shoulder, or arms. Older adults may complain of increased fatigue or shortness of breath.

54. D: Under the Healthy People 2030 initiatives, the target mean total cholesterol level for people age 20 and older is 186.4 mg/dL, which represents a 2.3% reduction from the 2013–2016 mean level of 190.9 mg/dL. Another initiative that focuses on cholesterol calls for an increase in the percentage of adults (at least 21 years of age) who have received treatment for high cholesterol to 54.9% from 44.9%.

55. C: For screening for cardiovascular risk in asymptomatic adults, a resting ECG is considered reasonable, and a fasting lipid profile (but not lipid parameters) is recommended. An echocardiogram may be considered for adults with hypertension but shows no benefit for nonhypertensive individuals. Genotype testing is not recommended. Another measure that is reasonable in asymptomatic adults is testing of HbA_{1C}. The ankle-brachial index may be used to assess asymptomatic adults with intermediate risk factors.

56. A: When utilizing the health belief model to help people to change behavior in order to manage chronic disease, the focus is on negative consequences of current behavior. Thus, if the goal is smoking cessation, the study materials may include pictures of blackened lungs and information about the adverse effects of smoking, such as increased risk of heart attack, stroke, and COPD. According to this theory, people will take action if they believe they can prevent negative consequences.

57. B: If a patient has received an automatic implantable cardioverter-defibrillator (AICD) in the left chest, instructions in the postoperative period should include avoiding lifting the left arm above the shoulder for 4 weeks as well as avoiding lifting more than 5 pounds with the arm; however, the arm can be used for daily activities. Although upper body exercises are usually restricted for up to 6 weeks, walking is acceptable unless otherwise contraindicated. Patients are usually advised only to call the physician with 1 shock if no ill effects are present, but to call EMS for more than 1 shock or if ill effects occur.

58. B: The primary purpose of wearing a LifeVest is to treat sudden cardiac arrest through defibrillation. The LifeVest, a wearable defibrillator, contains electrodes that monitor the heart rate and rhythm and detect abnormalities that lead to cardiac arrest. When cardiac arrest occurs, therapy pads in the back release electrode gel to promote effectiveness of shocks and to prevent burns, and then the pads provide a treatment shock, which may be repeated if the heart does not resume function.

59. A: The strongest predictor of a person's health status is literacy skills, with those with low literacy skills at increased risk of poor health outcomes. People with low literacy skills tend to be less knowledgeable about health issues and have higher rates of disease and hospitalization. Almost half of adults in the United States are classified as having low or moderate literacy skills, and this translates into low health literacy. Because of this, most educational material should be written at the fourth- to sixth-grade level.

60. C: If using the Modified Borg Scale for Perceived Dyspnea to evaluate endurance, severe dyspnea is indicated by a score of 7. The Modified Borg Scale for Perceived Dyspnea is as follows:

0: No dyspnea at all
0.5: Very, very slight dyspnea
1: Very mild dyspnea
2: Mild dyspnea
3: Moderate dyspnea and difficulty breathing
4: Somewhat severe dyspnea
6: Stronger or harder breathing
7: Severe dyspnea
8: More severe dyspnea
9: Extremely severe dyspnea
10: Dyspnea so severe unable to continue activity

61. B: When conducting the 6-minute walk test, an indication that the test should be stopped immediately is if the patient complains of leg cramps. Other indications for stopping the test include severe dyspnea (although some mild to moderate dyspnea is tolerable), chest pain, staggering gait (risk of fall), and diaphoresis (some increased perspiration is not cause for concern). The test should also be immediately discontinued if the patient appears ashen and pale (increasing risk of fainting).

62. A: When administering the NIH stroke scale to a patient, the cardiac/vascular nurse should conduct the test in the order items are listed, skipping no sections, and scoring while administering the test. The nurse should not go back and reassess items or adjust scoring, being sure to score what the patient is actually able to do rather than what the nurse believes the patient is capable of doing. Except for those items that require directions to the patient, the patient should not be coached in any way, such as by encouraging the patient to "try again."

63. D: An ankle-brachial index (ABI) of 0.85 (less than 0.9 is diagnostic) indicates peripheral arterial disease (PAD), with a score of 0.5–0.8 indicating moderate PAD and less than 0.5 indicating severe PAD. The normal range is from 1.0–1.4, with scores higher than that indicating non-compressible calcification, most common in older adults or those with diabetes. The ABI should be calculated (to 2 decimal places) separately for the right and left sides, as circulatory impairment may be more pronounced on one side.

64. C: The Pain Assessment in Advanced Dementia (PAINAD) scale evaluates 5 parameters: (1) respirations (rapid, labored hyperventilation, Cheyne-Stokes), (2) vocalization (quiet speech, moaning, crying), (3) facial expression (grimace, sad, frightened), (4) body language (tense, fetal position, pacing, fidgeting), and (5) consolability. The PAINAD scale is indicated for patients with impaired cognitive ability or the inability to verbalize the extent of pain. The patient should be observed carefully for nonverbal behaviors that are indicative of discomfort.

65. B: According to the ACC/AHA guidelines on the assessment of cardiac risk, the primary focus is on the lifetime risk for atherosclerotic cardiovascular disease (ASCVD). ASCVD is assessed based on the patient's age, gender, ethnic/racial background, systolic blood pressure, use of antihypertensives, diabetic status, smoking status, total cholesterol, and HDL cholesterol. Preventive measures for those at risk focus on blood cholesterol levels, obesity, and lifestyle management.

66. C: The Quality of Well-Being Self-Administered (QWB-SA) scale assesses a period of 3 days (the days prior to the test) rather than the 6 days in the original QWB in order to improve patient recall. The QWB-SA comprises 5 sections: chronic health problems, acute physical and mental symptoms, mobility, physical activity, and social activity. While the test is self-administered and can be completed in about 10 minutes, the scoring is weighted and somewhat complicated.

67. A: Out of the 15 questions posed on the Short-Form Geriatric Depression Scale (GDS) the minimum number of "yes" answers that indicate the patient is experiencing depression is 6 (more than 5). The GDS is self-administered and appropriate for older adults with normal cognition; however, the questionnaire may also be administered verbally to patients with mild to moderate cognitive impairment as long as they are aware enough to understand and respond to the questions.

68. D: The complementary therapy that is likely to be the most effective for a patient with sinus tachycardia is meditation. Sinus tachycardia is often associated with stress and anxiety; methods that help the patient to relax, such as meditation, relaxation, visualization exercises, and even yoga, may prove helpful. Some people find aromatherapy relaxing, but herbal medicines should be avoided as some may have adverse effects or may not be compatible with medications.

69. C: The apex of the heart, the point of maximum impulse, can usually be auscultated at the left fifth intercostal space, about 8–9 cm lateral to the mid-sternal line or slightly medial to the mid-clavicular line. The normal adult heart is approximately 12.5 cm in length and 9 cm at its widest point but may enlarge with cardiomyopathy or heart failure. The top of the heart lies at the second intercostal space with the heart extending downward to the fifth intercostal space.

70. D: The five phases of the normal cardiac cycle are:

1. Isovolumetric ventricular contraction: Ventricular depolarization results in increased ventricular tension, causing the mitral and tricuspid valves and the aortic and pulmonic valves to remain closed.
2. Ventricular ejection: Aortic and pulmonic valves open, and ventricles eject blood.
3. Isovolumetric relaxation: All valves are closed, and the atria fill with blood (atrial diastole).
4. Ventricular filling: Pressure in the atria causes the mitral and tricuspid valves to open, filling the ventricles (70% capacity).
5. Atrial systole: Atrial systole and late ventricular diastole supply the remaining 30% of the blood.

71. A: The four key functions of cardiac cells are:

- Automaticity (electrical property): Cells (pacemaker) are able to generate an electrical impulse. This is the most important function related to the cardiac rhythm.
- Excitability (electrical property): Cells are able to respond to the electrical impulse.
- Conductivity (electrical property): Cells are able to transmit the electrical impulse to other cells.
- Contractility (mechanical property): Cells are able to contract in response to an electrical impulse.

72. B: According to the Society for Vascular Nursing clinical practice guideline for carotid artery stenting, the antiplatelet therapy that is recommended pre-surgically is a combination of aspirin and clopidogrel. Both drugs should be administered to the patient for at least 24 hours prior to surgery and should continue up to 5 days after surgery. These drugs have different mechanisms of blocking activation of platelets, which is induced by the surgical procedure, so the antiplatelet therapy is critical to maintain patency of the stent.

73. C: If, when conducting a physical examination, the cardiac/vascular nurse finds the patient's BP is elevated to 170/88 mmHg and P is 92 bpm, the nurse should repeat the BP and P in 5 minutes to determine if the spike is due to "white coat" anxiety, a common situation. The BP and P often decrease after the patient has had a period of time to relax. BP should also be taken on both arms.

74. C: An S3 heart sound that occurs immediately after S2 over the mitral area is an indication of left ventricular noncompliance. The S3 heart sound, also referred to as a ventricular gallop, is a low-pitched heart sound that follows the rhythm of the word "Kentucky." The sound is most often heard during early to mid-diastole. If the right ventricle is noncompliant, the sound occurs in the tricuspid area. The S3 sound may be a normal variation in a child or adult younger than 30 years, but it is usually associated with a disorder for those older than 30 years.

75. B: The normal range for a patient's pulse pressure is 30–50 mmHg. The pulse pressure is calculated from the patient's blood pressure. The diastolic value is subtracted from the systolic value. Thus, if the BP is 140/90 mmHg, 140 minus 90 equals 50 mmHg. Increased pulse pressure may occur with increased stroke volume and decreased peripheral vascular resistance. Decreased pulse pressure may occur with mitral or aortic stenosis, peripheral vascular constriction, and decreased stroke volume.

76. A: When assessing a patient's peripheral perfusion with the patient lying flat in supine position, before assisting the patient to sit up and dangle the legs, the nurse should elevate one of the patient's legs 12 inches above the heart for 60 seconds. As soon as the patient sits up, the nurse should compare the color of the legs. The leg that was elevated should appear slightly paler than the other, but color should return in about 10 seconds, with venous refill in about 15 seconds. With arterial insufficiency, the return of color and venous refilling may be delayed, or the return color may appear mottled.

77. B: Capillary refill time of the finger nailbeds should not take more than 2 seconds. To assess capillary refill time, the nailbed should be firmly compressed for 5 seconds and then released and observed for return to color, noting the time required in seconds. If the capillary refill is delayed, this indicates impaired circulation, which may indicate low cardiac output and/or arterial insufficiency. The capillary refill time should be assessed on both the right and the left sides.

78. D: When assessing jugular venous distention, the patient should be positioned with the head elevated to about 45° while lying supine because, in a normal patient, jugular venous distention only occurs when the patient is lying flat. The nurse should locate the internal jugular vein, using care to distinguish it from the carotid artery. The nurse should note the highest point where pulsations can be observed. The distance in centimeters from the sternal notch to the highest point should be recorded. Jugular venous distention is present if the distance is more than 3–4 cm.

79. A: If a patient's finger capillary refill time is 7 seconds (prolonged) and blanching of the finger is followed by cyanosis and then erythema (red, white, and blue signs) before the color returns to normal, these findings are consistent with Raynaud syndrome, which results in vasoconstriction of the arterioles of the hands and/or feet. Initially, often only one or two fingertips are involved in the disease, but eventually all of the fingers and the distal palm are affected. Patients must avoid exposure to cold and smoking, as these may trigger vasoconstriction.

80. C: A patient with jugular venous distention that is more pronounced on inspiration and who complains of chest pain and exhibits hepatosplenomegaly, ascites, and peripheral edema should be assessed for pericardial friction rub because these signs and symptoms are associated with chronic constrictive pericarditis, which results in fibrosis of the pericardium. This fibrosis restricts ventricular filling, decreasing both cardiac output and stroke volume. Venous congestion is generally present systemically, resulting in peripheral edema, ascites, and hepatosplenomegaly.

81. B: The cardiac protein that is most specific to myocardial damage is troponin I because it is found only in the myocardium. Troponin T is also found in the myocardium but is found in skeletal muscle as well, so levels may elevate with muscle damage. Likewise, myoglobin is found in both skeletal muscle and the myocardium. Creatine kinase-MB is also found specifically in the myocardium, but it is less specific to myocardial damage than troponin I.

82. A: The cardiac protein that is expected to elevate first after an acute myocardial infarction is myoglobin, which is found in both skeletal muscle and the myocardium, so it is not specific to the heart (resulting in false positives). Following an MI, the myoglobin level increases in 2–4 hours, peaking in 8–12 hours, and returning to normal value (undetectable) within 12–30 hours (usually 24–30). Myoglobin level may be used to determine the advisability of thrombolytic therapy or emergent angioplasty within 6 hours of an MI.

83. C: The PLAC and LDL tests are used to predict the risk of coronary artery disease. When heart disease is present, macrophages increase production of lipoprotein-associated phospholipase A_2, and the PLAC test measures this enzyme. If the PLAC test shows increased levels and the LDL test is less than 130 mg/dL, then the individual has up to three times the risk of those without these findings. The higher the PLAC test and the lower the LDL level, the higher the risk of coronary artery disease.

84. D: If a patient has impaired kidney function and is receiving low-molecular-weight heparin (LMWH), the test most indicated to monitor heparin therapy is anti-Xa. While LMWH does not usually require monitoring, in the presence of kidney disease, levels may increase because of impaired excretion. Anti-Xa can be used to monitor both LMWH and unfractionated heparin, although the activated partial thromboplastin time (aPTT) is more commonly used for unfractionated heparin.

85. B: Following a cardiac arrest, the treatment most indicated to prevent neurological injury in unconscious survivors is therapeutic hypothermia. The patient should be placed in therapeutic hypothermia as soon as possible (within 2 hours of return of spontaneous circulation) and cooled to 32–34 °C and kept at this temperature for 12–24 hours before slowly being raised to normal body temperature. Studies indicate that survival rates are higher for patients receiving therapeutic hypothermia, and neurological impairment is less severe.

86. A: If an outpatient was prescribed a beta-blocker for exertional angina and calls to report that he has seen no relief in 48 hours, the cardiac/vascular nurse should advise the patient to expect the medication to take one to two weeks to begin to work. Beta-blockers are used for exertional angina because they decrease the physiologic response to exercise that usually results in increased heart rate and systolic blood pressure, so there is less myocardial oxygen demand.

87. A: Following a patient's myocardial infarction, the cardiac/vascular nurse needs to help the patient and family members understand:

- Limitations: physical activity/mobility parameters, pacing of activities
- Improvement potential: short-term and long-term expectations regarding return to health and previous level of activities
- Precautions: activities to avoid, signs and symptoms that require intervention, the correct method for taking medications (such as nitroglycerin)

The cardiac/vascular nurse should review these factors before the patient begins an activity program.

88. D: The responsibility for being a change agent in an organization should fall on all personnel because all staff members may be able to identify positive changes within their jobs or scopes of practice that will improve services or processes. Too often, staff members expect change to occur from the top down, but change from the bottom up is often more meaningful because it derives from those who are better able to assess the need for change.

89. A: In the role of preceptor for a graduate student, the cardiac/vascular nurse should expect the primary preceptor role to be to supervise and guide the student. Preceptorship is usually a time-limited arrangement, often lasting for a semester or for a student's rotation through a unit rather than an ongoing relationship, such as occurs with mentoring. The preceptor may only observe the student or may participate in care, depending on the established model, but it is important that the preceptor plan enough time in his or her work schedule to accommodate the student's needs.

90. B: When utilizing the SBAR method for hand-off, the information that should be conveyed for each element includes:

- S (Situation): identifying information, such as name, age, diagnosis, and physician
- B (Background): brief medical history, review of current treatments and lab results, physical status (VS, pain level), special needs, comorbidities, educational needs, and discharge plans
- A (Assessment): review of systems and any lines, tubes, or drains as well as explaining tasks that have been completed and those that still need completion, including future plans
- R (Recommendations): review of current care plan, including all medications, treatments, precautions, and wound care

91. B: While all of these are possible, the most likely explanation is that that patient is anxious. Some nonverbal behaviors are self-comforting, such as rubbing the hands together, licking the lips, and clasping the arms about the chest in a self-protective manner; these behaviors are often employed subconsciously as a reaction to stress and anxiety. Additionally, patients who are anxious may "tune out," such as by staring at something (such as the painting on the wall), and may not process information well during these times.

92. A: If a patient states, "I'm probably not going to survive this operation," and there is a good chance that the patient's assumption is correct, then the best response is to acknowledge the patient's statement without obliterating all hope: "It's a dangerous operation, but your surgeon is very skilled." The will to live is a strong force, and the nurse needs to support that as much as possible. Both "I'm sorry, but you are right" and "Do you have any last wishes that you want me to convey?" may suggest to the patient that the surgery is futile. "What makes you feel that way?" is simply avoiding the real issue.

93. C: The drug that is commonly used for a patient with a hypertensive emergency and acute heart failure is sodium nitroprusside, given per IV infusion (0.25–10.0 mcg/kg/min, usually beginning with 0.3 mcg/kg/min) with immediate onset of action and duration of one to two minutes. BP should be monitored every 5 minutes initially and then every 15 minutes. Nicardipine hydrochloride and labetalol hydrochloride are contraindicated with acute heart failure, and esmolol hydrochloride is indicated for SVT and post-operative (aortic dissection) tachycardia/hypertension.

94. D: The most common complication after endovascular aneurysm repair (EVAR) of abdominal aortic aneurysm is an endoleak, which occurs in up to 20–25% of patients and increases risk of rupture. While some leaks occur in the first month after surgery, leaks have been recorded as late as seven years after surgery. Other less common complications include local wound infection or hematoma (up to 10%), injury to the access artery (up to 3%), spinal ischemia (very rare), colonic ischemia (up to 3%), renal artery occlusion (less than 5%), and graft infection (up to 1%).

95. C: If the cardiac/vascular nurse finds in documenting in the electronic health record (EHR) that coded entries for some common signs and symptoms encountered in cardiac care are missing, the best solution is to request that information services add additional codes. EHRs almost always require some modification to meet the workflow and demands of different units, and while making free text entries places the information in the EHR, the data cannot be mined for analytical purposes.

96. A: If a patient is to be discharged with a number of medications and needs to check vital signs daily and have weekly blood tests, the patient may feel overwhelmed, so the most therapeutic response is one that acknowledges the problem and provides some solution: "Let's talk about this" (acknowledges the patient's concerns) "and work out a schedule together" (provides a collaborative solution). Engaging the patient in the process is more effective than simply giving advice ("You should. . .), agreeing ("You are right"), or using clichés ("Don't worry").

97. C: Most medical assistance programs, such as those that provide drugs at low or no cost to patients, are available to patients based on income. While requirements may vary according to the drug or manufacturer, income that is equal to or lower than the federal poverty level is the most common requirement. Patients can query drug companies directly, utilize a search engine, or use a patient assistance database, such as RxAssist.org, which allows searches by brand name, generic name, or drug company. For example, searching for generic drugs will render a list of all companies providing the drug and online applications.

98. B: If the cardiac/vascular nurse notes that a patient with a prosthetic heart valve has developed scattered petechiae on the body and splinter hemorrhages in the nail beds, the cardiac/vascular nurse should suspect infectious endocarditis. Other common immunologic manifestations include Osler's nodes (red swollen lesions with white centers on pads of fingers or toes, thighs, and palms of hands or soles of feet), Janeway lesions (purple non-tender 1–5 mm lesions on arms, legs, and palms of hands and soles of feet), conjunctival petechiae, and Roth's spots (small white spots in retina).

99. B: If an elderly Native American patient had been treated by tribal healers prior to hospitalization and is suspicious and uncooperative, the best solution is probably to ask healers to participate in treatment, as the patient likely has more faith in the healers than in Western medicine, and the rituals involved in healing ceremonies may be very comforting. The hospital should accommodate the needs of the healers as much as possible but should know if any herbs or other ingredients are used by the healers and, if so, whether they are acceptable.

100. C: If a patient tells a cardiac/vascular nurse something of a personal nature in confidence, the nurse should maintain confidentiality, according to HIPAA regulations, even if the patient has died. Information that a patient shares that is unrelated to the patient's condition or treatment, such as the fact that the patient's daughter was not her husband's, should not be divulged to others, including family members, or documented in the patient's records because this would also violate confidentiality.

101. B: In most states, advance directives are not legally binding and may be overridden by family members because health care providers are reluctant to stop treatment if family members insist the treatment be provided. Therefore, in most cases, the best advice is to encourage patients to discuss the matter with their families and to let the families know their wishes so that, if the issue arises, the families can make informed decisions based on what the patients want.

102. A: If a patient recovering from insertion of a pacemaker because of bradycardia related to heart block tells the cardiac/vascular nurse that she worries about living with cardiac disease and needs more information, the best referral is probably to the Mended Hearts. Mended Hearts provides educational resources and support groups for patients and families living with heart disease and offers peer-to-peer support programs for hospital visits, online support materials, and phone contact.

103. D: The primary purpose of risk management is to anticipate problems (such as potential civil suits related to negligence or malpractice) and to resolve them. Risk management evaluates and prioritizes risks as well as addresses them with the ultimate aim of reducing liability to an organization. If the potential for liability is present (such as if a patient falls and is injured), then personnel may meet with the family directly. Risk management is also active in planning insurance needs and ensuring adequate personnel, security, and safety policies.

104. C: If the nurse comes into a room in the cardiac care unit and finds the two daughters of the nonresponsive patient loudly arguing, the best response is to acknowledge there is a problem and seek to help resolve it: "Let's sit down together and talk about this." Sometimes, a third person acting as a mediator can help family members who are in disagreement express their feelings and concerns and arrive at a solution.

105. B: If the wife of a patient who is doing poorly has started spending hours in the hospital chapel praying and states that she believes God will save her husband, according to Kübler-Ross's five stages of grief, the stage of grief that the wife is probably undergoing is bargaining. These stages include:

Denial	People resist information or seem stunned, unable to comprehend.
Anger	People may express anger inwardly or outwardly, blaming themselves or others.
Bargaining	People utilize if-then thinking processes, appeal to God, or change doctors.
Depression	People become tearful, sad, and withdrawn.
Acceptance	People can accept the outcome with less pain and less preoccupation.

106. A: If, when monitoring a patient's telemetry, the cardiac/vascular nurse notes that the mean arterial pressure (MAP) has dropped from 70 to 55 mmHg, the nurse's immediate response should be to administer oxygen and notify the physician because an MAP greater than 60 mmHg is necessary for adequate perfusion of the internal organs. MAP is calculated with the systolic and diastolic blood pressure values:

$$\text{MAP} = \frac{\text{Diastole} \times 2 + \text{Systole}}{3}$$

107. B: If a patient who is a Jehovah's Witness is to undergo emergent angiography and angioplasty, the most important religion-related question to ask the patient is if she will accept blood products. While it is generally against the beliefs of the Jehovah's Witnesses to accept blood products, this does not necessarily hold true for all members. According to their religious beliefs, Jehovah's Witnesses can undergo surgery, take medications, and take fractions derived from blood, such as albumin and immune globulins.

108. A: The approach most commonly used for transcatheter aortic valve replacement (TAVR) is transfemoral. This procedure is generally limited to patients who are at high operable risk or are not candidates for traditional open-heart approaches. The bovine valve, supported by a metal stent, is inserted via a balloon catheter and guided into the heart and positioned inside of the aortic valve. Then the balloon is inflated, securing the valve. The transapical and transaortic approaches both require external incisions and may be utilized for patients with peripheral arterial disease that precludes the transfemoral approach.

109. C: While informed consent is critical, even when a patient has been fully apprised of a procedure and all of the elements required for informed consent, the patient still may not cognitively process the information, especially if the patient is confused, weak, or frightened. The nurse should immediately call the physician and report the patient's misconception so that the physician can ensure that the patient is informed and fully understands the procedure.

110. B: If a patient qualifies for home health care under Medicare (Original), Medicare will pay the agency a fee based on the patient's condition for an "episode of care," which is a period of 60 days. Services that Medicare will cover include part-time or intermittent skilled nursing care, physical therapy, occupational therapy, speech-language pathology services, medical social services, and medical supplies, such as dressing supplies. Durable medical equipment is paid for separately by Medicare (usually 80% of approved cost).

111. A: The purpose of Home and Community-Based Services (HCBS) programs provided through Medicaid is to maintain patients in their home environments rather than nursing homes for as long as possible. Under the HCBS services, patients may be eligible for a number of different services, such as home health care and personal care services as well as some services that are not usually provided by Medicaid or Medicare, including adult day services, transportation assistance, and home modifications.

112. A: There are five "rights" of delegation: the right person, right task, right circumstance, right direction/communication, and right supervision. All of the individuals available are technically qualified to provide personal care; therefore, the right person is not the primary consideration. In this case the decision to delegate to the CNA with 5 years of experience in the unit is an example of the right circumstance. Even though the CNA has less formal education than the LVN, the LVN has no work experience in the unit and therefore may not be able to efficiently collect the materials and provide care to an already anxious patient. Familiarity with the unit will allow the CNA with 6 years of experience to provide patient-centered care that the circumstance requires. The CNA's 5 years of actual work experience should have provided the RN with a good estimation of the person's skills, and it is the responsibility of the RN to make a judgment about who is best suited to provide care.

113. D: If the cardiac/vascular nurse believes that a procedure can be effectively shortened without any compromise in quality, the next step should be to write a formal proposal for change and submit it to the appropriate authority, which may vary from one institution to another. Changing procedures is not always an easy task because procedures should be based on best evidence and are usually included in procedure manuals and training, so any change, even a minor modification, may require multiple responses—such as changing training procedures, educating staff, and changing procedure manuals.

114. D: The type of coping strategy that a patient is exhibiting when the patient constantly asks questions and utilizes Internet searches to obtain information about all treatments and medications is trying to maintain control. In this case, knowledge is power. Other coping strategies that patients and families employ include using social support (such as family and friends), using spiritual support (prayer, meditation, spiritual advisor), accepting the situation (dealing with the situation realistically), and being optimistic (expecting the best).

115. B: If, when users of the new electronic health record (EHR) were evaluated, the cardiac/vascular nurse was the only nurse on the unit with no errors, while many others were struggling to utilize the new system correctly, the cardiac/vascular nurse should offer to serve as a resource person. Assisting others in a professional capacity and ensuring that care is documented properly is part of maintaining and promoting a healthy work environment.

116. A: Following a carotid endarterectomy, if a patient exhibits bradycardia, weak tone of voice, and dysphagia, the most likely reason is trauma to the superior laryngeal vagus nerve (X), which lies very close to the carotid artery and can be easily traumatized during surgery or affected by edema. Bradycardia must be treated promptly because it can lead to cerebral ischemia and neurological impairment. Vagal stimulation may also result in reflex hypotension in the first few hours after surgery.

117. B: When assessing cardiovascular function, the two most important symptoms to question the patient about are pain and shortness of breath. If the patient has pain, it is important to determine where the pain occurs and whether it radiates, precipitating factors, pain characteristics (burning, tight, sharp, dull), and factors that relieve the pain. If the patient has shortness of breath, the cardiac/vascular nurse should ask when it begins, how long it persists, if it occurs at night, and if the patient has also experienced coughing.

118. D: The task that can be delegated to unlicensed assistive personnel (UAP) is emptying a urinary catheter bag and measuring the urine. Some tasks can only be completed by registered nurses, and these include determining interventions needed in the plan of care, checking a patient's vital signs during an episode of chest pain (although UAP may take routine vital signs), and identifying goals related to the nursing diagnosis. Only RNs may develop nursing diagnoses, validate assessment data, and evaluate the effectiveness of care.

119. C: The type of defense mechanism that a patient is utilizing when the patient refuses to get out of bed or attend to any self-care (e.g., bathing, brushing teeth) and leaves decision-making to the patient's spouse is regression, which is reverting to an earlier developmental stage when trying to cope with stress. During periods of regression, patients may seem unable to make decisions or tell someone else to make the decisions for them. Patients may seem withdrawn and depressed.

120. A: If the cardiac/vascular nurse is caring for a close friend of a nurse on another unit and the nurse asks about the results of the patient's laboratory tests, the best response is, "I'm sorry, I can't give you that information." Most nurses are aware of HIPAA regulations, so reminding the nurse is probably not necessary, but sometimes nurses want others to overlook the regulations when they are seeking information; however, only those involved in the patient's care can legally have access to the patient's records.

121. D: According to the Eighth Report of the Joint National Committee on Prevention, Detection, Evaluation, and Treatment of High Blood Pressure, blood pressure should be treated pharmacologically in the general population when blood pressure is 140/90 mmHg or higher in patients younger than 60 and when blood pressure is 150/90 mmHg or higher when the patient is 60 and older. If the patient has diabetes in addition to hypertension, pharmacologic treatment should begin when blood pressure is 140/90 mmHg or higher in any age.

122. A: The diagnoses should be prioritized (first to last) in the following order for interventions:

1. Acute pain related to myocardial infarction: This has first priority because pain control is a physiological need and can be usually be treated rapidly with appropriate analgesia.
2. Risk for fluid volume excess related to heart failure: This is also a physiological need but requires observation over a more extended period of time.
3. Imbalanced nutrition, more than body requirements: This is not an acute need because it requires dietary assessment and counseling and well as lifestyle changes.
4. Risk for ineffective coping: This is a security need that requires assessment and education over an extended period of time.

123. B: A normal ejection fraction (EF), which is dependent on cardiac output, is 55–70%, representing the percentage of blood expelled from the ventricles during a contraction. Because this patient's EF is quite low at 33%, a realistic outcome for treatment is to improve the EF to at least 40%, which is still below normal but poses less risk to the patient. An EF below 35% increases the risk of potentially life-threatening dysrhythmias and cardiac arrest and may require an implantable cardioverter defibrillator.

124. D: If a patient has been prescribed simvastatin, lovastatin, or atorvastatin for high cholesterol, grapefruit juice should be limited to less than 1 quart daily. Grapefruit juice can result in increased blood levels of the drugs and increased adverse effects. Licorice should be avoided with digoxin because the combination may result in digoxin toxicity. Cranberry products should not be taken while on warfarin. Milk does not pose a problem with cardiovascular medications.

125. C: Patients taking loop and/or thiazide diuretics should be routinely monitored for potassium levels because both types of diuretics increase the secretion of potassium because they inhibit sodium and chloride reabsorption. The normal range for potassium levels is 3.5–5.5 mEq/L; hypokalemia is defined as a serum potassium level less than 3.5 mEq/L. The critical value for potassium is less than 2.5 mEq/L. Symptoms of hypokalemia include weakness, lethargy, nausea and vomiting, paresthesia, muscle cramps, tetany, hypotension, and dysrhythmias. ECG changes include PVCs and flattened T waves.

126. A: Beta-blockers should not be used for treatment for patients with severe asthma. Some of the newer classes of beta-blockers (such as metoprolol) are specific to beta-1 adrenergic receptors and may be utilized for patients with mild to moderate asthma if they do not respond adequately to other classes of medication, but they should be monitored closely. Beta-blockers may cause cough-variant asthma in patients without previous history of asthma. Patients on beta-blockers should be cautioned to never abruptly stop the medication, as it may result in angina, dysrhythmias, or heart attack.

127. C: If a patient receiving digoxin 0.25 mg daily had a recent serum digoxin level of 1.8 ng/mL (normal therapeutic levels are 0.5–2.0 ng/mL) but is exhibiting a pulse rate of 56 bpm with occasional dysrhythmia, the cardiac/vascular nurse should withhold the medication (pulse below 60 bpm) and begin ECG monitoring (dysrhythmia). Patients may develop digoxin toxicity even with serum digoxin levels within normal range. The serum digoxin level and potassium levels should be checked, and potassium should be administered if hypokalemia is present. Anti-dysrhythmic medications and digoxin immune Fab may be administered, depending on the patient's condition.

128. D: The Unna boot is contraindicated for patients who have nonambulatory status. Because the boot depends on the pumping action of the muscles to reduce edema, the boot must be removed if the patient is unable to ambulate. The Unna boot is used to treat venous stasis and venous ulcers but is contraindicated if the ulcers are infected or if phlebitis is present. The Unna boot is a gauze wrap impregnated with zinc oxide, glycerin, or gelatin. The gauze should be applied distally to proximally without tension and be left open to dry or covered with self-adherent wrap. The Unna boot may be changed twice weekly to every other week.

129. B: The primary reason to begin cardiac rehabilitation while the patient is still in the acute hospital is to prevent the negative results of deconditioning. Ideally, rehabilitation should begin 3–5 days after an MI or cardiac surgery and should include educating the patient about her condition and diagnostic tests as well as outlining the type of cardiac rehabilitation she will undergo and any limitations she will have on discharge. The patient should be introduced to the behavior modification (such as smoking cessation, diet, and exercise) that will be needed.

130. D: In an older adult, key indications of coronary artery disease are fatigue and dyspnea. While adults often experience angina, the sympathetic response in older adults may be muted, so they may be essentially asymptomatic or complain of general malaise. Additionally, as patients begin to experience fatigue and dyspnea, they often moderate their activities so that they are less likely to have overt symptoms. Lack of angina in older adults should not rule out the possibility of coronary artery disease.

131. C: A patient with hypertrophic cardiomyopathy (also known as idiopathic cardiomyopathy) is especially at risk for sudden cardiac death. Hypertrophic cardiomyopathy is characterized by hypertrophy of the left ventricle and thickening of the left side of the intraventricular septum. The left ventricle becomes increasingly noncompliant and cannot relax during filling, so left atrial and pulmonary venous pressures increase, resulting in dyspnea. Complications include pulmonary hypertension, heart failure, ventricular arrhythmias, and sudden cardiac death.

132. A: The ECG changes that are common to myocardial injury and myocardial infarction include ST-segment elevation and T-wave inversion, so onset of these changes should signal the need for further testing, such as cardiac enzymes and proteins. With myocardial ischemia, the first stage of heart damage, ST-segment depression and T-wave inversion are common. In the second stage, when the ischemia is prolonged and damage occurs, then ST-segment elevation is evident. In the third stage, myocardial infarction, the first change may be tall T waves, but these become inverted, and ST-segment elevation occurs as the hours pass.

133. C: An absolute contraindication to thrombolytic use for a myocardial infarction is suspected aortic dissection. Other absolute contraindications include previous intracranial hemorrhage, vascular cerebral lesions, malignant intracranial neoplasm, ischemic stroke within 3 months, active bleeding (other than menses), history of significant head trauma or surgery in the preceding 3 months, intracranial/intraspinal surgery within 2 months, and severe hypertension (uncontrolled and unresponsive). Relative contraindications include internal bleeding within 2–4 weeks, current anticoagulation therapy with warfarin (INR at least 2–3), and history of chronic, severe, poorly controlled hypertension.

134. A: Apixaban is an anticoagulant (direct factor Xa inhibitor) that is used to prevent clots with atrial fibrillation. Apixaban interacts with a number of different drugs, so a patient's medications should be scrutinized to make sure they are safe to use with the drug. In this case, paroxetine (an SSRI) may increase the risk of bleeding if taken with apixaban. Other drugs that should be avoided are SNRIs, aspirin, NSAIDs, azole antifungals (such as ketoconazole), phenobarbital, phenytoin, and St. John's wort.

135. B: According to the AHA/ACC/HRS guideline for the management of patients with atrial fibrillation, the recommended antithrombotic therapy for patients with mechanical heart valves and atrial fibrillation is warfarin. The target INR should be maintained at 2–3 or 2.5–3.5, depending on the type of prosthesis and the location. The INR should be monitored weekly during initiation of treatment and at least monthly when the INR has stabilized.

136. D: While various formulas and computerized calculations are used to accurately calculate the corrected QT (cQT) interval, which is the interval between the beginning of the Q wave and the end of the T wave, one method to estimate the cQT is based on the standardized cQT: ≤0.42 seconds at 60 bpm. In order to estimate, 0.02 seconds is subtracted from 0.42 seconds for every 10 bpm that the patient's heart rate exceeds 60 bpm. Since the patient's heart rate is 90 bpm (30 beats higher), then $0.02 \times 3 = 0.06$ seconds less, or 0.36 seconds.

137. D: When using a radial pressure device to promote hemostasis after an arterial blood draw, once the pressure device is applied, it should be left in place initially for 30 minutes to ensure that bleeding does not occur. It's important when applying the device to ensure that the compression pad (and gauze pad, if used) is positioned directly over the puncture site, that the minimal pressure needed to achieve hemostasis is utilized, and that the radial pulse distal to the compression pad is palpable.

138. A: If a patient must have an IV inserted and blood tests but states that she is terrified of needles and may faint, the best course of action is to ask the patient what might help to relieve her anxiety before deciding on any other intervention. In some cases, a patient with a phobic fear of needles may be comforted by having a family member present. Patients are not often reassured by being told the procedure is not painful because it is not necessarily the pain that they are afraid of, and they may be too tense to take deep breaths and relax. If time permits, antianxiety medications may help patients to cope better.

139. C: According to the AHA/ACC/HRS guideline for the management of patients with atrial fibrillation, in order to successfully maintain sinus rhythm after cardioversion for atrial fibrillation, the atrial fibrillation should have had a duration of less than 6 months. Over time, the frequency of episodes of atrial fibrillation tends to progress from paroxysmal atrial fibrillation/tachycardia to persistent as remodeling of the heart's electrical system occurs. When fibrillation/tachycardia is persistent, it is more difficult to treat.

140. B: When a patient is undergoing cardiac rehabilitation, a measure that may be used for the behavioral outcome domain is the exercise regimen, including the frequency and the type of exercises. The clinical domain would measure heart rate, percent of body fat, body weight, and other clinical data, such as oxygen saturation. The health domain would measure the quality of life as well as morbidity and mortality. The service domain would measure satisfaction of stakeholders (patients, clinicians), and the economic outcome domain would measure things related to costs, such as length of stay, number of emergency visits, and costs of care.

141. C: First-degree relatives of patients with familial dilated cardiomyopathy should be screened for the disorder with serial echocardiography every 3–5 years so that LV function and size can be evaluated. Patients and family members may also consider genetic testing and counseling. Up to 35% of patients diagnosed with idiopathic dilated cardiomyopathy actually have the familial type, so patients diagnosed with idiopathic cardiomyopathy should tell first-degree relatives so they can discuss the need for testing with their clinicians.

142. A: When assessing the cardiovascular system of an older adult, the cardiac/vascular nurse should expect posterior displacement of the apical pulse because of cardiac hypertrophy. Other differences include altered landmarks for assessment and distant heart sounds related to kyphosis. Because of increasing rigidity of the valves associated with calcification or stenosis, aortic or mitral systolic murmurs may be present without cardiovascular pathology. Systolic BP tends to increase in older adults, while the diastolic pressure may increase or decrease, and widened pulse pressure may be observed.

143. D: If, when assessing a patient, the cardiac/vascular nurse notes central cyanosis, this likely indicates a reduction in oxygen saturation, usually associated with inadequate oxygenation of the blood because of cardiopulmonary disease, such as congenital defect or chronic obstructive pulmonary disease (COPD). A reduction in blood flow may result in peripheral cyanosis as well as cyanosis of the ears and nose. If clubbed fingers are observed, these usually result from prolonged reduction in oxygen saturation.

144. B: If a patient is having a pharmacologic echocardiogram with IV dipyridamole and develops shortness of breath and dizziness, the medication the cardiac/vascular nurse should expect to administer to relieve the adverse effects is aminophylline. The medication should be available during the procedure, which involves giving increasing dosages of dipyridamole at 5-minute intervals. The patient's vital signs should be monitored during the test and after until they return to baseline, and the patient should be observed for signs of distress.

145. D: The DASH eating plan to control hypertension is based on about 2000 calories per day, so patients who are overweight or obese may need to modify the diet to lower caloric intake. The daily diet includes 6–8 servings of grains, 4–5 servings of vegetable, 4–5 servings of fruit, 2–3 servings of low/fat-free milk products, 6 ounces or less of protein source (lean meat, poultry, eggs), and 2–3 servings of fat and oils. In addition, patients should have 4–5 servings of nuts, seed, and legumes per week and 5 or fewer servings of sweets and added sugars.

146. C: If a patient is prescribed metoprolol for control of supraventricular tachycardia and hypertension, the cardiac/vascular nurse should advise the patient to avoid abruptly stopping the medication, as this can lead to rebound hypertension and worsen symptoms of ischemic heart disease—and may even cause a myocardial infarction. If the patient must discontinue the medication, the patient needs to decrease the dosages slowly under the advice of a physician. Beta-blockers may be less effective for African Americans than for those of other ethnic backgrounds.

147. A: For health promotion, primary, secondary, and tertiary prevention methods are needed:

- Primary: aims to prevent a disease before it actually occurs, often through public campaigns, such as those that encourage exercise, smoking cessation, and a healthy diet
- Secondary: aims to prevent further deterioration for those who already have a disease, such as by early detection through screening programs or advising low-dose aspirin for those at risk
- Tertiary: aims to help patients control their disease and manage disease effectively through such interventions as cardiac rehabilitation programs and support groups

148. B: If a patient shows nonverbal indications of pain (e.g., tense, withdrawn, frowning, holding her chest) as well as increased respiratory and heart rate but describes pain on a 1-to-10 scale as "2," the cardiac/vascular nurse should ask the patient about pain in another way, such as "mild, moderate, or severe." Although the use of the 1-to-10 scale is ubiquitous in health care, it is not commonly used or understood in some cultures, and many people are unsure how to rate pain.

149. A: Patients may exhibit ineffective coping in response to serious illness, recent changes in health status, or personal vulnerability. Patients may exhibit ineffective coping in a number of ways, such as by the inability to make decisions, poor concentration, emotional tension, general irritability, or chronic depression. Interventions include establishing a trusting relationship, allowing the patient to express concerns, exploring the patient's feelings about physical changes, assessing the patient's problem-solving skills, and assisting the patient to recognize personal strengths.

150. C: If a fellow nurse for whom the cardiac/vascular nurse is serving as a mentor gave a patient the wrong dose of a medication, the best response is, "What did you learn from this experience?" This response helps the nurse to focus on avoiding future errors. Medication errors, while they can have serious consequences, are rarely the result of intentional negligence, and a punitive approach ("You are lucky you didn't get fired!") or lecturing ("I hope you learned how important double-checking is") serves little purpose. The mentor should also avoid excessive sympathy ("You poor thing…").

Practice Test #2

1. According to the ACCP Antithrombotic Therapy and Prevention of Thrombosis, the cardiovascular event prophylaxis that should be used for patients with asymptomatic peripheral arterial disease is:

a. ASA 75–100 mg daily or clopidogrel 75 mg daily
b. ASA 75–100 mg daily
c. ASA 75–100 mg daily and clopidogrel 75 mg daily
d. ASA 75–100 mg daily and warfarin

2. A patient with a permanent implanted pacemaker complains of fatigue, palpitations, and dizziness. Examination shows the patient has jugular venous distention and pulsations in the neck as well as hypotension. The most likely cause is:

a. Pacemaker system infection
b. Lead perforation
c. Twiddler syndrome
d. Pacemaker syndrome

3. When calculating the QT interval, a correction (cQT) should only be made if the heart rate is at or above:

a. 80 bpm
b. 70 bpm
c. 60 bpm
d. 50 bpm

4. What is the primary difference between a POLST form and an advance directive?

a. There is no essential difference.
b. The POLST form is intended only for those with serious life-threatening illness.
c. The POLST form is intended only for those without serious life-threatening illness.
d. The advance directive is intended for those with more serious illness.

5. In order to be a true interdisciplinary team, which of the following is a critical element?

a. Collective goal
b. Strong leader
c. Individual goals
d. Hierarchical structure

6. A patient with irregular SVT has received a 6-mg bolus of IV adenosine after failing to respond to verapamil. What electrocardiographic change does the cardiac/vascular nurse anticipate may occur with the adenosine?

a. Cardiac arrest
b. Atrial flutter
c. Atrial fibrillation
d. Transient asystole

7. A patient with severe heart failure exhibits a Cheyne-Stokes pattern of breathing during sleep, usually resulting in:

a. Insomnia
b. Hypothermia
c. Hypoxemia
d. Hypercapnia

8. If a patient develops a rapid heart rate after administration of nitroglycerine for angina, the most likely cause is:

a. Increased cardiac ischemia
b. Reflex tachycardia
c. Atrial fibrillation
d. Myocardial infarction

9. According to Bandura, self-efficacy is the most important factor in adherence. Which of the four sources of self-efficacy is most important?

a. Learning from modeling
b. Experience with mastery
c. Physiologic cues
d. Verbal/social persuasion

10. Which cardiac disorder puts the patient most at risk for sudden cardiac death?

a. Right ventricular dysfunction
b. Left ventricular dysfunction
c. Right atrial dysfunction
d. Left atrial dysfunction

11. According to ACC/AHA/HRS Guidelines for the Management of Patients with Atrial Fibrillation, the target INR for patients receiving warfarin for atrial fibrillation is usually:

a. 0.5–1.0
b. 1–2
c. 2–3
d. 3–4

12. The precordial leads in a 12-lead ECG record electrical activity in the:

a. Frontal plane
b. Sagittal plane
c. Median plane
d. Horizontal plane

13. When carrying out health promotion activities regarding risk factors for coronary heart disease, the cardiac/vascular nurse recognizes that the four primary risk factors are (1) hypercholesterolemia, (2) hypertension, (3) physical inactivity, and (4):

a. Family history of cardiovascular disease
b. Obesity
c. Cigarette smoking
d. Anxiety

14. When a patient is undergoing therapeutic hypothermia after cardiac arrest, the patient must be maintained above what temperature, as an absolute rule?

a. 28 °C
b. 30 °C
c. 32 °C
d. 34 °C

15. A patient complains of sudden onset of sharp stabbing substernal pain that radiates to the neck and left shoulder. The pain increases with inspiration and with lying in supine position but is alleviated by sitting upright and leaning forward. These symptoms are consistent with:

a. Pericarditis
b. Acute myocardial infarction
c. Dissecting aortic aneurysm
d. Angina pectoris

16. Based on the NYHA classification of patients with heart disease, the cardiac/vascular nurse would expect that a person classified as functional class III would exhibit:

a. Symptoms at rest
b. No symptoms with ordinary physical activities
c. Symptoms with ordinary physical activities
d. Symptoms with less than ordinary physical activities

17. At which of these American Heart Association (AHA) heart failure stages does a patient's heart failure symptoms disrupt daily life and often lead to hospitalization?

a. Stage A
b. Stage B
c. Stage C
d. Stage D

18. According to the ACCP Antithrombotic Therapy and Prevention of Thrombosis, which antithrombotic/prophylactic therapy should a patient with atrial fibrillation and a CHADS2 score of 2 receive during the first three to six months after angioplasty with placement of a drug-eluting stent?

a. ASA and clopidogrel
b. Warfarin only
c. ASA, clopidogrel, and warfarin
d. Warfarin and ASA

19. If a patient with heart disease performs at Bruce protocol exercise level of 9 minutes on a treadmill (stage 3, 14% grade at 3.4 mph), how may METS of activity can the patient be expected to perform?

a. 7
b. 10
c. 13
d. 15

20. The Patient Self-Determination Act (1991) primarily supports which of the following ethical principles?

a. Autonomy
b. Justice
c. Beneficence
d. Nonmaleficence

21. When educating a patient about managing medications and monitoring vital signs and health conditions, the biggest problem is likely to be the patient's ability to:

a. Comprehend information.
b. Store information.
c. Retrieve stored information.
d. Respond to information.

22. The first stage in the learning process for adults is:

a. Paying attention
b. Processing information through the senses
c. Responding to information
d. Encoding information

23. When a cardiac/vascular nurse is serving as a mentor, a central concept of Bandura's social learning theory that is applicable is:

a. Reflection
b. Role modeling
c. Reward
d. Transference

24. According to Maslow's hierarchy of needs, which of the following nursing diagnoses has priority?

a. Risk for falls
b. Risk for ineffective coping
c. Compromised family coping
d. Ineffective airway clearance

25. When prioritizing a cardiac patient's learning needs according to mandatory, desirable, and non-essential needs, which of the following would be classified as a mandatory learning need?

a. Elements of a low fat/low sodium diet
b. Pathological changes in the patient's cardiovascular system
c. Signs and symptoms of heart failure
d. Rationale for exercise regimen

26. Which of the following statements by a patient taking nitroglycerine suggests a need for more education?

a. "I leave the pills out on the counter, so they are easy to get at."
b. "The sublingual wafers burn when I put them under my tongue."
c. "I know I shouldn't take Viagra with nitroglycerine."
d. "I should call 911 if I get no relief after the third dose."

27. A patient is to receive discharge education about his medications and treatments shortly after learning that he has an aortic aneurysm but is a poor candidate for surgery. Which of the following types of readiness to learn is likely to be the most impacted?

a. Physical
b. Emotional
c. Experiential
d. Knowledge

28. Which of the following is a characteristic of a field-independent learner?

a. Provides self-directed goals
b. Is easily affected by criticism
c. Places emphasis on facts over principles
d. Prefers experiential learning

29. When conducting a series of two-hour workshops as part of a cardiac rehabilitation program for a group of eight patients, the cardiac/vascular nurse notes that one patient routinely becomes restless after about 15 minutes and excuses herself to go to the bathroom, moves about the room, or seems to "space out." The most likely reason is:

a. Boredom
b. Discomfort
c. Anxiety
d. Short attention span

30. In motivational interviewing, responding to patients is primarily through:

a. Reflective listening
b. Change talk
c. Normalizing
d. Decisional balancing

31. What is the biggest obstacle to long-term management of cardiovascular disease?

a. Cost
b. Patient debility
c. Non-adherence
d. Social/peer pressure

32. The primary purpose of the Patient Learning Needs Scale is to:

a. Determine rehabilitation needs.
b. Evaluate the patient's knowledge of his/her disease.
c. Plan education for discharge.
d. Assess the patient's learning style.

33. When considering developmental stages, which of the following is a normative age-graded influence?

a. Divorce
b. Serious injury in a moving vehicle accident
c. The September 11, 2001 terrorist attack
d. Menopause

34. For percutaneous transluminal coronary angioplasty (PTCA) to be considered successful, residual stenosis after balloon inflation should be less than:

a. 20%
b. 30%
c. 40%
d. 50%

35. Considering barriers to learning, changes in fluid intelligence associated with aging may result in:

a. Diminishing of stimulus
b. Decreased test anxiety
c. Faster processing time
d. Altered perception of time

36. Which of the following goals of older adults is most likely to increase their motivation to learn?

a. Independence
b. Social acceptability
c. Personal resources
d. Coping mechanisms

37. In order to compensate for patients' hearing losses, teaching strategies may include:

a. Using a high-pitched voice
b. Speaking more loudly than usual
c. Exaggerating lip movements when talking
d. Using word speed of 140 words per minute or less

38. When assessing the ankle-brachial index, at what angle should the Doppler wand be held in relation to the skin?

a. 10°
b. 30°
c. 45°
d. 90°

39. The six-minute walk test is generally done over a distance of how many meters?

a. 20
b. 30
c. 40
d. 50

40. If, during the clinical interview, a patient states she is allergic to a medication, the initial response of the cardiac/vascular nurse should be to:

a. Ask what type of reaction the patient had.
b. Document the allergy and move to the next item of the interview.
c. Ask the patient if it was a true allergy or adverse response.
d. Ask how long the patient has had the allergy.

41. According to ACC/AHA guidelines, if a patient is admitted with angina, and the ECG indicates an ST-segment elevation myocardial infarction (STEMI), the next step should generally be:

a. To wait for results of cardiac markers
b. Reperfusion therapy
c. To observe patient for further symptoms
d. Coronary artery bypass graft

42. A patient's oxygen saturation per pulse oximetry has been stable at 95–96% but suddenly drops to 85% even though the patient does not appear to be in distress. The first action of the cardiac/vascular nurse should be to:

a. Administer oxygen.
b. Reposition the pulse oximeter.
c. Call an emergency response.
d. Notify the MD.

43. When using the FICA (faith and belief – importance and influence – community – address in care) rubric for a spiritual assessment of a patient, "community" refers to:

a. Neighborhood of residence
b. People of the same ethnic group
c. Religious/support group, such as church, synagogue, or mosque
d. City or town of residence

44. If a patient reports that he experienced an episode of severe chest pain seven days previously and has had recurrent chest pain, dyspnea, and weakness since that time, the most appropriate cardiac marker to determine if the patient experienced a myocardial infarction is probably:

a. Myoglobin
b. CK-MB
c. Troponin I
d. Troponin T

45. What is a normal value of troponin I in an adult (over age 18)?

a. Less than 0.04 ng/mL
b. Greater than 0.1 ng/mL
c. 0.2 ng/mL
d. Greater than 0.2 ng/mL

46. Which of the following B-type natriuretic peptide (BNP) levels is consistent with heart failure, requiring light limitation of physical activity?

a. 50 pg/mL
b. 100 pg/mL
c. 375 pg/mL
d. 650 pg/mL

47. In an ECG tracing, which of the following represents ventricular depolarization?

a. QRS complex
b. ST-segment
c. PQR complex
d. PQRST complex

48. When monitoring cardiac telemetry, the cardiac/vascular nurse notes a prominent U wave, which may represent:

a. Normal variation
b. Hyperkalemia
c. Hypokalemia
d. Hypocalcemia

49. If a patient complains of angina, the cardiac/vascular nurse recognizes that this usually means that one or more coronary arteries are occluded by at least:

a. 50%
b. 70%
c. 85%
d. 90%

50. According to the Venous Thromboembolism Risk Factor Assessment, which of the following factors poses the greatest risk?

a. Age 60–74
b. History of previous major surgery
c. Current chemotherapy
d. Hip fracture within the previous month

51. If the cardiac/vascular nurse is to assess a patient who speaks no English with the NIH stroke scale, but the scale is not available in the patient's language, the best course of action is to:

a. Wait until a medical translator can be located.
b. Ask a family member to translate.
c. Conduct the assessment in English, using pantomime and gestures.
d. Document that the stroke scale could not be completed.

52. If the cardiac/vascular nurse notes slight edema of the right foot and ankle and the patient complains of pain on palpation in the calf area with dorsiflexion of the foot, the nurse should suspect:

a. Deep vein thrombosis
b. Strained muscle
c. Varicose veins
d. Injury to Achilles tendon

53. The complementary/alternative therapy that should generally be avoided in patients with cardiovascular disease is:

a. Acupuncture
b. Aromatherapy
c. St. John's wort
d. Meditation

54. When stratifying patients who are to undergo exercise for cardiac rehabilitation according to risk of cardiac events, which of the following would pose the highest degree of risk?

a. Exercise-induced ST-segment depression less than 2 mm from baseline
b. Functional capacity less than 5 METS
c. Angina with activity level greater than 7 METS
d. Rest ejection fraction less than 40%

55. When teaching a patient how to use a Holter monitor, the patient repeatedly says, "Can I see that?" and "Show me...". This suggests that the best teaching aids may be:

a. Written explanations
b. Pictures and diagrams
c. Audiotapes
d. Flash cards

56. A patient with heart failure has a nursing diagnosis of decreased cardiac output. When documenting the care plan, an appropriate Nursing Outcome Classification (NOC) for this diagnosis is:

a. Cardiac pump effectiveness
b. Activity tolerance
c. Compliance behavior
d. Electrolyte and acid/base balance

57. According to the ACCF/AHA Guideline for the Management of Heart Failure, patients who are at Stage A of risk for heart failure because of hypertension and diabetes mellitus but without structural heart disease or heart failure symptoms should be treated with a(n):

a. Beta-blocker
b. Diuretic
c. Aldosterone antagonist
d. ACE inhibitor or ARB

58. According to the ACCF/AHA Guideline for the Management of Heart Failure, the definition of heart failure with borderline ejection fraction is demonstrated by an ejection fraction of:

a. ≤40%
b. 41–49%
c. 50–70%
d. >75%

59. When a patient is at rest, what percentage of the body's total blood volume is generally contained in the heart and pulmonary bed?

a. 15–25%
b. 25–50%
c. 50–60%
d. 60–80%

60. Hypoxia that is caused by decreased blood flow to the tissues is classified as:

a. Hypoxic hypoxia
b. Ischemic hypoxia
c. Anemic hypoxia
d. Histotoxic hypoxia

61. A coronary atherosclerotic lesion that is 25 mm in length with angulated segments of more than 90° is classified according to ACC/AHA guidelines as Class:

a. A
b. B
c. C
d. D

62. Which of the following anticoagulants is an antagonist of vitamin K?

a. Warfarin
b. Aspirin
c. Unfractionated heparin
d. Low-molecular-weight heparin

63. If a patient taking a cardiac glycoside (digoxin) is to also to take a calcium channel blocker (verapamil), the dosage of the cardiac glycoside should be:

a. Increased 25%
b. Decreased 25%
c. Increased 50%
d. Decreased 50%

64. Which of the following medications should be discontinued for a minimum of 48 hours before cardioversion?

a. Digoxin
b. Warfarin
c. Cardizem
d. Insulin

65. If a patient has undergone fibrinolytic therapy per accelerated infusion of alteplase 100 mg for an acute myocardial infarction and shows 20% reduction in ST elevation after 90 minutes, the cardiac/vascular nurse anticipates:

a. Further monitoring
b. Additional thrombolysis
c. Angiography/rescue percutaneous coronary intervention (PCI)
d. Administration of fondaparinux

66. If a patient complains loudly about her physician and states that the physician is incompetent, which of the following is the best response?

a. "The physician is very knowledgeable and competent."
b. "You should be less critical about your doctor."
c. "Do you want another physician?"
d. "You're concerned that you are not getting better."

67. The cardiac/vascular nurse is providing treatment for an older Japanese female patient, but the patient does not make eye contact and responds very quietly. This behavior probably represents:

a. Unhappiness with care
b. Fear of the nurse
c. Respect for the nurse
d. Major depression

68. For a patient about to be discharged after implantation of a pacemaker, the role of the faith community nurse is primarily to:

a. Pray with the patient and provide spiritual guidance.
b. Provide patient care within the home environment.
c. Assess the patient's needs and make referrals.
d. Arrange visits with spiritual advisors, such as pastors.

69. An appropriate role of the home health nurse for a patient being discharged from an acute care hospital after a myocardial infarction with PCI (angioplasty) is to:

a. Transport the patient to and from appointments.
b. Monitor vital signs and treatment adherence.
c. Assist the patient to hire a housekeeper.
d. Administer daily oral medications to the patient.

70. The cardiac/vascular nurse is participating in a health fair at the local shopping mall. Which of the following may be the most appropriate activity to attract visitors to the nurse's booth?

a. Place large posters above the booth.
b. Give out brochures about services.
c. Provide a monitor with a video about health screening.
d. Offer a service, such as a BP check.

71. According to the ACC/AHA Guideline on the Assessment of Cardiovascular Risk, race- and gender-specific Pooled Cohort Equations should be used to predict 10-year risk for a first hard atherosclerotic cardiovascular disease (ASCVD) event for:

a. All non-Hispanic men and women, ages 40–79
b. All non-Hispanic men and women, ages 20–79
c. All non-African American and non-Hispanic men and women, ages 40–79
d. All non-African American and non-Hispanic men and women, ages 20–79

72. Exercise electrography is recommended for cardiovascular screening for coronary artery disease for:

a. Symptomatic adults
b. All adults 65 years or older
c. All adults 40 years or older
d. All adults 70 years or older

73. When conducting a sleep assessment for a patient with heart failure, the cardiac/vascular nurse recognizes that the two cardinal signs of sleep apnea are:

a. Snoring and increased BMI
b. Snoring and daytime sleepiness
c. Insomnia and daytime sleepiness
d. Snoring and dry, sore throat

74. When conducting an assessment of a patient's retina, the cardiac/vascular nurse notes a silver wire artery. This usually indicates:

a. Diabetic retinopathy
b. Increased intracranial pressure
c. Inflammation
d. Hypertension

75. If the abdominojugular reflex shows a rise in the jugular venous pressure of 4 cm throughout pressure application, this indicates:

a. Right atrial failure
b. Left atrial failure
c. Right ventricular failure
d. Left ventricular failure

76. When measuring and documenting paradoxical blood pressure, the first documented systolic sound is that heard on:

a. Expiration
b. Inspiration
c. Both inspiration and expiration
d. Either inspiration or expiration

77. A summation gallop can be heard on auscultation of the heart in the presence of:

a. Cardiac failure with tachycardia
b. Aortic stenosis
c. Myocardial infarction
d. Impaired systolic function

78. What is the reference range for the cardiac marker CK-MB?

a. 0–5%
b. 12–20%
c. 32–36%
d. 95–100%

79. If the echocardiogram indicates increased left ventricular intracavity dimension and decreased ventricular wall movements, these findings are consistent with:

a. Restrictive cardiomyopathy
b. Hypertrophic cardiomyopathy
c. Dilated cardiomyopathy
d. Arrhythmogenic right ventricular dysplasia (ARVD)

80. Which of the following diagnostic procedures is most indicated for suspected aortic dissection in a stable patient?

a. Transthoracic echocardiography
b. CT scan
c. MRI
d. X-ray

81. When estimating the heart rate from an ECG strip, the cardiac/vascular nurse should begin by counting the number of:

a. QRS complexes in a 6-second strip
b. ST-segments in a 6-second strip
c. R waves in a 6-second strip
d. R-R intervals in a 6-second strip

82. Which of the following would make a patient ineligible for a left ventricular assist device (LVAD)?

a. Age over 65 years
b. Lack of social/family support
c. Ineligibility for transplant
d. Ejection fraction under 25%

83. If a patient is to be discharged after a pacemaker is implanted in the chest, the patient should be advised to avoid:

a. The distributor of a gas-operated engine
b. Microwave ovens
c. Walking through anti-theft security gates
d. Electric hand tools

84. If a patient is wearing a LifeVest and hears the device sound an alarm but feels all right, the patient should:

a. Lie down in preparation for the shock.
b. Press buttons to stop the shock sequence.
c. Remove the LifeVest immediately.
d. Disconnect the monitor from the garment.

85. When teaching a patient to manage wound care prior to discharge following CABG, the cardiac/vascular nurse utilizes teach-back by:

a. Demonstrating the procedure to the patient repeatedly
b. Asking the patient to teach another patient the procedure
c. Demonstrating and then testing the patient on the procedure
d. Asking the patient to demonstrate and explain the procedure

86. Under Healthy People 2030, the amount of stroke-related deaths should decrease from 37.1 per 100,000 in 2018, to:

a. 20 per 100,000
b. 25.5 per 100,000
c. 30.2 per 100,000
d. 33.4 per 100,000

87. An appropriate expectation of a volunteer visitor to patients in their homes is to:

a. Provide wound care.
b. Monitor medications.
c. Provide social interaction.
d. Assist with housekeeping.

88. The purpose of paratransit services is to:

a. Provide transportation to patients from requested address to destination.
b. Evaluate a patient's need for transportation devices, such as wheelchairs.
c. Provide taxi service to patients who are unable to drive independently.
d. Provide funds to patients to use to pay for their transportation needs.

89. A patient with coronary artery disease wants to quit smoking but is unable to attend smoking cessation classes because of health problems and lack of transportation. Which of the following is the best resource that the cardiac/vascular nurse can provide?

a. 1-800-QUIT-NOW
b. Visit from a non-smoker
c. Video about stopping smoking
d. Brochure on stopping smoking

90. In order to participate in a pharmaceutical assistance program, the patient must:

a. Apply through Medicare.
b. Apply through the insurance company.
c. Ask a physician to apply.
d. Apply directly to the manufacturer.

91. A patient with no family wants to ensure that her advance directive is respected. The cardiac/vascular nurse should recommend that the patient:

a. Give copies to all her physicians and healthcare providers.
b. Carry a copy in her purse.
c. Ask the local hospital to keep a copy on file.
d. Place a copy on her refrigerator door.

92. What is the primary purpose for using the SBAR (situation-background-assessment-recommendation) method for hand-off procedures?

a. Reducing liability
b. Speeding hand-off procedures
c. Reducing staffing needs
d. Promoting patient safety

93. If a patient has developed a life-threatening arrhythmia and the cardiac/vascular nurse notifies the physician on call but, when the physician arrives, the nurse notes that the physician smells of alcohol and has slurred speech, the nurse should:

a. Immediately notify a supervisor.
b. Confront the physician.
c. Report the physician to the medical board.
d. Ask another physician to intervene.

94. A patient confides to the cardiac/vascular nurse that the antihypertensive medication he has been taking has resulted in increasing impotence, so he has decreased the dosage and frequency. Which of the following is the best response?

a. "You must take the medication as it's prescribed."
b. "You need to talk to the physician about changing the medication or dosage."
c. "That is a terrible idea."
d. "As long as your blood pressure is stable, that is all right."

95. If the cardiac/vascular nurse directs an unlicensed assistive personnel (UAP) to conduct a bladder scan of a patient but discovers later that the UAP had only observed but never actually done the procedure and, thus, interpreted the scan incorrectly, the nurse should:

a. Report the UAP to the supervisor.
b. Reprimand the UAP for endangering the patient.
c. Ignore the situation as no ultimate harm came to the patient.
d. Take responsibility for improper delegation.

96. The cardiac/vascular nurse notes that a patient seems angry and upset after the doctor has left. Which of the following is an example of therapeutic communication?

a. "Try not to worry. Everything will be ok."
b. "You should talk about what's bothering you."
c. "Why are you so upset?"
d. "Is there anything you'd like to talk about?

97. In order to successfully manage conflict in the workplace, management must first:

a. Develop a conflict management system.
b. Recognize the existence of conflict.
c. Maintain open communication.
d. Survey staff members about conflict.

98. Which of the following patients with aortic stenosis would be an acceptable candidate for transcatheter aortic valve replacement (TAVR)?

a. A patient who is also eligible for open-chest surgery
b. A patient who cannot tolerate anticoagulants
c. A patient with comorbid endocarditis
d. A patient who is not a candidate for open-chest surgery

99. If an 18-year-old Jehovah's Witness patient begins to hemorrhage following open-heart surgery and signs a consent for blood transfusions but his parents insist he cannot have transfusions and state they will sue if the cardiac/vascular nurse administers a transfusion, the nurse should:

a. Administer the blood transfusion.
b. Withhold the blood transfusion.
c. Consult risk management.
d. Ask the physician to speak with the parents.

100. Which of the following is a criterion for endovascular thoracic aortic aneurysm repair?

a. Patient has Marfan disease-associated thoracic aortic aneurysm.
b. Patient has ascending thoracic aortic aneurysm.
c. Aneurysm is at least double the size of the adjacent aorta.
d. Aneurysm is less than 5 cm in diameter.

101. Elective cardioversion is synchronized with the ECG, and the current is delivered during the:

a. QRS complex
b. R-R interval
c. T wave
d. ST segment

102. According to the ACC/AHA Focused Update of the Guideline for the Management of Patients with Peripheral Artery Disease, which of the following is recommended to reduce risk of MI, stroke, or vascular death in patients with atherosclerotic lower extremity peripheral arterial disease?

a. Clopidogrel 150 mg daily
b. Warfarin
c. Unfractionated heparin
d. ASA 75 mg to 325 mg daily

103. According to the Eighth Report of the Joint National Committee on Prevention, Detection, Evaluation, and Treatment of High Blood Pressure, when lifestyle changes alone do not control high blood pressure, which of the following is NOT an initial drug of choice to treat hypertension?

a. Beta-blocker
b. Thiazide diuretic
c. Angiotensin receptor blocker
d. ACE inhibitor

104. To ensure correct fit of a blood pressure cuff and correct readings, how much of the arm should the cuff bladder encircle?

a. 100%
b. 80%
c. 60%
d. 50%

105. If a patient has high blood pressure readings during visits with clinicians but reports lower blood pressure readings at home, the best solution is to:

a. Calibrate home BP device.
b. Treat according to home BP readings.
c. Treat according to clinical BP readings.
d. Conduct ambulatory blood pressure monitoring (ABPM).

106. According to the Eighth Report of the Joint National Committee on Prevention, Detection, Evaluation, and Treatment of High Blood Pressure, what is the maximum number of ounces of wine per day that is acceptable for a male patient?

a. 5 ounces
b. 10 ounces
c. 12 ounces
d. 16 ounces

107. Which of the following drugs is recommended as the preferred initial antihypertensive agent for preventing complications of hypertension?

a. Thiazide diuretic
b. Beta-blocker
c. Calcium channel blocker
d. ACE inhibitor

108. A Middle Eastern patient admitted for heart failure is found to have a number of annular ecchymotic regions up and down the back with some evidence of hematomas and small lacerations. What is the most likely reason?

a. Physical abuse
b. Wet cupping
c. Coining
d. Gridding

109. If a patient exhibits resistant hypertension, what is the first thing to evaluate before changing medications?

a. Kidney function
b. Drug interactions
c. Adherence to treatment regimen
d. Accuracy of blood pressure readings

110. A patient who has been hospitalized for a week asks the cardiac/vascular nurse, who lives in the patient's neighborhood, to go by the patient's house and water her plants after work. The nurse should:

a. Do as the patient requests.
b. Offer to help the patient contact a friend or neighbor.
c. Advise the patient that the request is inappropriate.
d. Tell the patient that the nurse doesn't have time.

111. If a cardiac/vascular nurse suspects that a patient is not adhering to lifestyle modifications and is lying about doing so and telephones the patient's brother for information about the patient without telling the patient, this is an example of:

a. A HIPAA violation
b. A professional boundary violation
c. Holistic care
d. Malpractice

112. Because of changing demographics and increased costs of medical care, the cardiac/vascular nurse expects that future medical care will likely place more emphasis on:

a. Alternative treatments
b. Long-term care
c. Acute care
d. Preventive care

113. If a cardiac/vascular nurse conducts literature research and proposes a different approach to patient triage based on evidence-based practices, and the practice improves efficiency and the quality of patient care, the nurse could be best described as a(n):

a. Leader
b. Innovator
c. Change agent
d. Team player

114. According to the diffusion of innovation theory, when innovative change is proposed, which adopter category is likely to include the smallest number of individuals?

a. Late majority
b. Laggards
c. Early adopters
d. Innovators

115. When promoting change within an organization, the cardiac/vascular nurse should recognize that the primary means by which staff members interpret and understand the dynamics of change is per:

a. Informal communication with peers
b. Top-down communication
c. Formal information channels
d. Personal research

116. If interdisciplinary team meetings are continuously disrupted by two members who disagree with each other during brainstorming, which of the following techniques may be most useful in resolving the conflict during the meetings?

a. Delphi survey technique
b. Nominal group technique (NGT)
c. Task list
d. Prioritization matrix

117. In an interdisciplinary team, one member frequently and effusively praises one of the other members. This is an example of a member trying to gain influence over another through:

a. Assertiveness
b. Exchange
c. Ingratiation
d. Rationality

118. A patient who has a very poor prognosis appears quite cheerful and talks about her plans for a long vacation in Europe after she leaves the hospital. The primary defense mechanism that the patient is using is:

a. Reaction formation
b. Denial
c. Dissociation
d. Repression

119. If an illegal Mexican immigrant without insurance is treated in the ED for a myocardial infarction, the best referral on discharge in most states is likely the:

a. Public health department
b. State Medicaid program
c. Mexican consulate
d. Free clinic, such as RotaCare

120. A physician has ordered an expensive new drug for a patient who has minimal insurance. If the patient tells the nurse that she cannot pay her child's college tuition and pay the medication costs, the cardiac/vascular nurse should first:

a. Discuss the situation with the physician.
b. Advise the patient that her health is most important.
c. Suggest the patient explore a pharmaceutical assistance program.
d. Tell the patient to ask the doctor to prescribe a different medication.

121. If a patient has a nursing diagnosis of extracellular fluid volume excess and one of the goals is to prevent specific manifestations of the extracellular fluid volume excess, which of the following are appropriate outcome criteria for this goal?

a. Signs and symptoms of extracellular fluid volume excess are noted at onset.
b. Patient's weight declines toward normal, and breathing sounds improve.
c. Patient denies orthopnea or dyspnea, and blood gases are normal.
d. Patient maintains normal weight and exhibits no S3, crackles, or peripheral edema.

122. The primary treatment focus for patients with dilated cardiomyopathy is:

a. Promoting activity
b. Controlling heart failure
c. Preparing for heart transplant
d. Preventing sudden death

123. When an elderly patient is to be removed from life support, his daughter complains loudly that her father was selfish and brought his illness on himself by refusing to cooperate with his physicians. The daughter's reaction is probably an expression of:

a. Grief
b. Family estrangement
c. Lack of caring
d. Lack of health literacy

124. A patient is awaiting surgical intervention for a dissecting aortic aneurysm. Prior to surgery, the patient's systolic BP should be maintained at:

a. 90–100 mmHg
b. 100–110 mmHg
c. 110–120 mmHg
d. 120–130 mmHg

125. If an ICD must be turned off for a procedure, the safest method is to:

a. Place a magnet over the ICD.
b. Program the ICD into OFF mode.
c. Surgically remove the ICD.
d. Carefully follow manufacturer's instructions.

126. Which of the following precautions is necessary for a patient with an implanted ICD?

a. Cell phone should be at least 6 inches away from ICD implantation site.
b. Patient should avoid all hand-held security detectors.
c. Patient should stand at least 6 feet away from arc welding equipment.
d. Patient should avoid driving for one year after implantation.

127. From the perspective of risk management, the best method to improve patient safety is probably:

a. Imposition of sanctions when patient safety is compromised
b. Better training for healthcare providers about patient safety
c. Reward system for compliance with patient safety measures
d. Improvement in staff:patient ratio

128. If a patient has suspected endocarditis, which of the following diagnostic tests are most indicated?

a. CT scan and blood cultures
b. MRI and blood cultures
c. CBC and ECG
d. Blood cultures and echocardiogram

129. When applying an Unna boot, the correct application is:

a. Wrap first layer from toes up to knee and second layer in reverse.
b. Wrap from the knee down toward the toes.
c. Wrap from toes up toward knee.
d. Apply inner wrap vertically and second wrap horizontally from toes to knee.

130. After application of a radial pressure device, if the cardiac/vascular nurse notes a small amount of blood oozing from the puncture site, the next step is to:

a. Remove the device and apply manual pressure.
b. Slowly increase the pressure until bleeding stops.
c. Remove the device and reapply to ensure proper site pressure.
d. Increase the pressure to the next number on the dial.

131. The primary cause of mitral stenosis in patients is:

a. Rheumatic fever
b. Endocarditis
c. Congenital abnormality
d. Malignant carcinoid syndrome

132. Following ethanol alcohol septal ablation in a patient with hypertrophic cardiomyopathy, the patient must be carefully monitored for:

a. Left bundle branch block
b. Atrial fibrillation
c. Supraventricular tachycardia
d. Right bundle branch block

133. According to the ACCP Antithrombotic Therapy and Prevention of Thrombosis, a patient with suspected recurrent lower extremity DVT should have which of the following initial diagnostic procedures?

a. Compression ultrasound
b. MRI
c. Venography
d. CT venography

134. Following a severe myocardial infarction, a patient is no longer able to walk six blocks to a subway station and has been utilizing taxi services to attend a cardiac rehabilitation program, but the patient states she may not be able to continue with rehabilitation because of the transportation expense. The cardiac/vascular nurse should advise the patient to:

a. Take the taxi only to and from the subway station.
b. Utilize an alternate service, such as Uber or Lyft.
c. Ask neighbors and friends if they can provide transportation.
d. Contact the public transportation authorities about paratransit services.

135. Which of the following congenital heart diseases pose low risk to the pregnant patient?

a. Cyanotic congenital heart disease
b. Aortic valve disease (unrepaired)
c. Small, unrepaired ventricular septal defect
d. Coarctation of the aorta

136. Although a Spanish-speaking Hispanic male being monitored in an outpatient clinic has set appointment times, the patient rarely arrives at the scheduled time, sometimes coming early but often arriving one to two hours late. The most likely reason is:

a. Lack of transportation
b. Lack of consideration of staff
c. Cultural perception of time
d. Inadequate English skills

137. Which of the following types of medications is less effective for African Americans than other ethnic groups?

a. Thiazide diuretics
b. ASAs
c. Calcium channel blockers
d. ACE inhibitors

138. If a patient is admitted to the cardiac care unit in hypertensive crisis with BP of 240/140 and is started on IV sodium nitroprusside, the initial treatment goal should be to reduce BP by:

a. 50%
b. 40%
c. 25%
d. 10%

139. When assisting a female patient with lifestyle management, the cardiac/vascular nurse notes that the patient's BMI is 31 kg/m^2 and her waist measurement is 39 inches. These findings would classify the patient as:

a. Overweight
b. Obese
c. Severely obese
d. Morbidly obese

140. When a patient is using the Borg Rating of Perceived Exertion (RPE) Scale (6-20) to rate the amount of effort an activity requires, walking slowly for a few minutes without problem is usually quantified as a:

a. 9
b. 11
c. 13
d. 15

141. Which of the following is an example of an isotonic activity?

a. Lifting
b. Carrying
c. Pushing
d. Walking

142. If a patient is admitted to the ED and reports no relief of chest pain after taking nitroglycerine three times at 5-minute intervals and the presumptive diagnosis is unstable angina or NSTEMI, the initial treatment should include oxygen and:

a. Beta-blocker
b. Unfractionated heparin
c. ASA
d. Warfarin

143. Which of the following ECG findings most suggest coronary ischemia?

a. ST-segment depression and T-wave inversion
b. ST-segment elevation and T-wave inversion
c. Hyper-acute T wave, ST-segment elevation, and T-wave inversion
d. ST-segment elevation and pathologic Q waves

144. Which of the following is a dysrhythmia characterized by a regular heart rate of 160 beats per minute with abnormally shaped P waves (that may be hidden in the preceding T waves) but with a normal PR interval and normal QRS complex?

a. Sinus tachycardia
b. Paroxysmal supraventricular tachycardia
c. Junctional dysrhythmia
d. Atrial flutter

145. The cardiac/vascular nurse would expect a patient being admitted for acute decompensated heart failure to present with:

a. Peripheral edema
b. Chest pain
c. Generalized erythema
d. Pulmonary edema

146. A pacemaker with the NBG code of VDD senses:

a. Both atria and ventricles but paces only ventricles
b. Only ventricles and paces only ventricles
c. Only ventricles but paces atria and ventricles
d. Only atria and paces only atria

147. Following radiofrequency ablation, the patient must be taught to monitor:

a. Daily weight
b. Fluid intake
c. Pulse
d. Sodium intake

148. If a patient's functional capacity allows for medium activity (3.5–5.0 METS), which work activity is allowable?

a. Plumbing
b. Shoveling
c. Mowing lawns
d. Digging ditches

149. According to Tong's criteria for decision-making in relation to the ethical principle of justice, which of the following criteria has priority?

a. Effort
b. Contribution
c. Merit
d. Need

150. The nurse notes physiological splitting of the S2 heart sound. This type of splitting results from:

a. Inspiration
b. Expiration
c. Electrical delay
d. Both inspiration and expiration

Answer Key and Explanations for Test #2

1. B: According to the ACCP Antithrombotic Therapy and Prevention of Thrombosis, the cardiovascular event prophylaxis that should be used for patients with asymptomatic peripheral arterial disease is ASA 75–100 mg daily only. This regimen has been shown to slightly reduce overall mortality over a 10-year period. The routine use of ASA also increases the risk of major bleeding, so the benefit of MI prevention must be balanced against the risk of bleeding.

2. D: If a patient with a permanent implanted pacemaker complains of fatigue, palpitations, and dizziness, and examination shows the patient has jugular venous distention and pulsations in the neck as well as hypotension, the most likely cause is pacemaker syndrome, which is inappropriate timing of atrial and ventricular contractions. Symptoms occur with VVI pacing, as the loss of AV synchrony can result in reflex vasodilation and hypotension. Resultant low cardiac output causes the fatigue and weakness as well as exertional dyspnea.

3. C: When calculating the QT interval, a correction (cQT) should only be made if the heart rate is at least 60 bpm because the formula for calculation is not accurate with slower pulses. The cQT is also difficult to assess if the heart rate is irregular because the QT interval varies according to heart rate. Different formulas and electronic calculators can be used to determine the cQT. The standardized cQT at 60 bpm is 0.42 seconds with an estimated cQT done by subtracting 0.02 seconds for each increase in heart rate of 10 bpm.

4. B: The primary difference between a POLST (physician orders for life-sustaining treatment paradigm) form and an advance directive is that the POLST form is intended only for patients with serious life-threatening illness, while everyone should complete an advance directive. The POLST form contains a medical order, such as DNR, so it must be filled out and completed by a clinician. POLST forms are not yet available in all states, and programs go by a variety of names.

5. A: In order to be a true interdisciplinary team, a critical element is a collective goal. Unless the group is working collectively, it may be a work group (in which people have individual goals and/or projects) or a pseudogroup (in which there is little focus or direction). Interdisciplinary teams should have stable membership so that the members can develop relationships over time. In a team, leadership roles may rotate because hierarchical structure is less important than working together.

6. D: If a patient receives a 6-mg bolus of IV adenosine after failing to respond to verapamil, the electrocardiographic change the cardiac/vascular nurse should anticipate is transient asystole. Adenosine is an unclassified antidysrhythmic that slows electrical conduction through the AV node. Because adenosine has a very short half-life of only 10 seconds, it is only administered as a rapid IV push, resulting in the asystole that persists for a few seconds. Because of its short half-life, other adverse effects are minimal.

7. C: If a patient with severe heart failure exhibits a Cheyne-Stokes pattern of breathing during sleep, this usually results in hypoxemia as periods of central apnea alternate with hyperpnea. These recurrent periods of hypoxemia may further damage a failing heart. Patients may exhibit decreased alertness during waking hours because of the frequent interruptions of sleep. Pulmonary congestion is common, reducing the stores of gas in the lungs so that changes in the ventilatory pattern have a greater effect than normal on blood gas values.

8. B: If a patient develops a rapid heart rate after administration of nitroglycerine for angina, the most likely cause is reflex tachycardia because of the sudden vasodilation and shift in fluids from the heart toward the systemic circulation. Baroreceptors in the myocardium sense this as a sudden loss of blood and increase the heart rate to compensate for the perceived blood loss. The tachycardia is short-lived, as the same baroreceptors sense that the blood volume is adequate and decrease the heart rate.

9. B: According to Bandura, self-efficacy is the most important factor in adherence, and experience with mastery, previous success at achieving goals, is the most important source of that self-efficacy. Patients who believe they can be successful are more likely to adhere to treatment regimens because they see the value in persistence. Other sources include learning from modeling (seeing others perform tasks successfully), physiologic cues (symptoms), and verbal/social persuasion (convincing others that they can be successful).

10. B: The cardiac disorder that puts the patient most at risk for sudden cardiac death is left ventricular dysfunction, especially with ejection fraction under 30% or with ventricular dysrhythmias following a myocardial infarction. Most cases of sudden cardiac death occur following myocardial infarction, and warning signs may be absent. Patients who are resuscitated are at increased risk of another episode of sudden cardiac death because of the electrical instability of the heart.

11. C: The target INR for patients receiving warfarin for atrial fibrillation is usually 2–3. The INR should be monitored weekly during initiation of therapy and at least monthly after levels have stabilized. If patients require withholding of warfarin for procedures, then patients with mechanical heart valves should receive bridging therapy with unfractionated heparin or low-molecular weight heparin, while those without mechanical heart valves should be evaluated on an individual basis to determine risk of adverse effects (such as stroke) during the period when warfarin is discontinued.

12. D: The precordial leads in a 12-lead ECG record electrical activity in the horizontal plane (anterior and posterior and right/left). The six precordial leads are placed on the chest, while the six limb leads are placed on the arms and legs, recording electrical activity in the frontal plane (up and down and right/left). If necessary, arm electrodes can be positioned on the shoulders and leg electrodes on the inferior rib cage without a significant change in signal.

13. C: When carrying out health promotion activities regarding risk factors for coronary heart disease, the cardiac/vascular nurse recognizes that the four primary risk factors are (1) hypercholesterolemia, (2) hypertension, (3) physical inactivity, and (4) cigarette smoking. Cigarette smoking is of primary concern because it interacts with hypercholesterolemia and hypertension to increase risk associated with those conditions. Smoking (especially the nicotine and carbon monoxide) accelerates atherosclerosis throughout the entire body, but this is of special concern in the coronary arteries.

14. B: When a patient is undergoing therapeutic hypothermia after cardiac arrest, the patient's temperature must be kept above 30 °C. The ideal range is between 32 and 34 °C for 12–24 hours before slowly warming to normal temperature. The target temperature is ordered by the physician, which is generally part of an order set that also includes parameters for the cooling, maintenance and rewarming phases. Medications for shivering are generally included in this order set, in addition to electrolyte replacement protocols and frequency of assessment and documentation. The patient's temperature must be closely monitored, generally by two mechanisms of internal temperature monitoring, such as a Foley catheter probe and a rectal probe. The risk of arrhythmias increases if the body core temperature falls to less than 30 °C, and the myocardium responds less effectively to medications and defibrillation. If the body temperature falls to less than 28 °C, the risk of ventricular fibrillation increases.

15. A: If a patient complains of sudden onset of sharp stabbing substernal pain that radiates to the neck and left shoulder, increasing with inspiration and with lying in supine position but alleviated by sitting upright and leaning forward, these symptoms are consistent with pericarditis. Patients may complain of dyspnea when lying flat and may appear anxious. Some may develop a dry cough. If pericarditis is constrictive, patients may develop peripheral edema.

16. D: Based on the NYHA classification of patients with heart disease, the cardiac/vascular nurse would expect that a person classified as functional class III would exhibit symptoms with less than ordinary physical activities. Patients with functional class III generally have no symptoms while at rest but begin to exhibit symptoms (such as dyspnea and/or chest pain) with less than ordinary physical activities.

17. D: With AHA Stage D heart failure, the patient is in what is considered 'advanced heart failure' with symptoms disrupting daily life and hospitalizations recurring. The AHA stages heart failure based on the disease progress and while the NYHA classifies heart failure based on how it limits physical activity.

18. C: According to the ACCP Antithrombotic Therapy and Prevention of Thrombosis, the antithrombotic/prophylactic therapy that a patient with atrial fibrillation and a CHADS2 score of 2 should receive during the first three to six months after coronary angioplasty with placement of a drug-eluting stent is triple therapy with warfarin, ASA, and clopidogrel. If patients have bare metal stents, then the triple treatment is given for one month after placement. Following these initial periods, patients are maintained on warfarin plus an antiplatelet drug.

19. B: If a patient with heart disease performs at Bruce protocol exercise level of 9 minutes on a treadmill (stage 3, 14% grade at 3.4 mph), the patient can be expected to perform at 10 METS. The Bruce protocol begins at 5 METS, with increased increments of grade and speed every 3 minutes, with each increase equivalent to an additional 2–3 METS. The duration of the total test is 21 minutes (7 stages), with the grade beginning at 10% and 1.7 mph (stage 1, 5 METS) and ending at 22% and 6 mph (20 METS).

20. A: The Patient Self-Determination Act (1991) primarily supports the ethical principle of autonomy. Under provisions of this act, healthcare institutions, such as hospitals and rehabilitation centers, are required to provide patients a written outline of decision-making rights (including the right to refuse treatment), inquire if the patient has an advance directive and document the status in the patient record, educate staff regarding advance directives, and avoid any discrimination against patients who do not have advance directives.

21. C: When educating a patient about managing medications and monitoring vital signs and health conditions, the biggest problem is likely to be the patient's ability to retrieve stored information. One of the primary tasks of information processing is to comprehend and process information so that it can be stored. If stored in short-term memory, information may only be retrieved within a few seconds to a few minutes, but even if stored in long-term memory, patients may have difficulty retrieving the information and responding to it.

22. A: The first stage (1) in the learning process for adults is paying attention. Patients are often in pain or distracted by health concerns; if they are unable to focus their attention, then learning is not likely to take place. The next stage (2) is processing information through the senses (auditory, visual, kinesthetic), followed by (3) encoding the information into short-term memory, where it is either lost or transmitted into long-term memory. The last stage (4) is responding to the information in a meaningful way, such as by application.

23. B: A central concept of Bandura's social learning theory is role modeling. Bandura believed that people learn by observing others, so the behavior that a cardiac/vascular nurse exhibits is of primary importance to others in the nurse's sphere of influence, such as the person that is being mentored. Another concept is that of vicarious reinforcement, that is whether or not the role model is validated or punished for the behavior the mentor exhibits because this may influence the behavior of the mentee.

24. D: According to Maslow's hierarchy of needs, physical needs have the highest priority, followed by safety needs, belonging and love needs, esteem needs, and lastly, self-actualization. Ineffective airway clearance poses the greatest physical risk and has first priority. Risk for falls, a safety concern, is the second priority. Because compromised family coping is an issue related to belonging and love, it is the third priority, with ineffective coping being the last priority because it is related to esteem and the perception of competence.

25. C: When prioritizing a cardiac patient's learning needs according to mandatory, desirable, and non-essential needs, a mandatory learning need is for the patient to learn the signs and symptoms of heart failure so that the patient is able to get help before the condition becomes life-threatening. Both the elements of a low fat/low sodium diet and the rational for an exercise regimen are desirable. While some patients may be interested in the pathological changes in the cardiovascular system, this is non-essential information.

26. A: Because nitroglycerine should be protected from light (maintained in original packaging or amber-colored glass container), the statement that suggests a patient needs more education is: "I leave the pills out on the counter, so they are easy to get at." Nitroglycerine tablets usually maintain potency for only three to six months, so they must be replaced on a regular schedule. Sublingual wafers should burn slightly. If they do not, then the wafers are likely outdated and have lost potency.

27. B: If a patient is to receive discharge education about his medications and treatments shortly after learning that he has an aortic aneurysm and is a poor candidate for surgery, the type of readiness to learn that is likely to be the most impacted is emotional readiness. If the patient is severely anxious or worried about his prognosis, then the patient may not absorb information, regardless of its importance, and there is often little time to allow the patient to recover, so the cardiac/vascular nurse must engage the patient in the learning process, such as by stressing health protective measures.

28. A: Field-independent learners view themselves as separate from others and tend to be less affected by criticism, peer pressure, or external feedback and prefer to provide self-directed goals and to organize material by themselves. They are more interested in applying general principles than focusing on facts. They often prefer lecture to discussion. Field-dependent learners, on the other hand, are easily affected by criticism, peer pressure, and external feedback and need external goals. They prefer organized facts to principles and discussion over lecture.

29. D: If, when conducting a series of two-hour workshops as part of a cardiac rehabilitation program for a group of eight patients, the cardiac/vascular nurse notes that one patient routinely becomes restless after about 15 minutes and excuses herself to go to the bathroom, moves about the room, or seems to "space out," the most likely reason is a short attention span. When teaching patients, it's important to vary presentations at least every 10–15 minutes, such as by providing a period for questions and answers.

30. A: In motivational interviewing, responding to patients is primarily through reflective listening. With this technique, the cardiac/vascular nurse listens to what the patient has to say and then paraphrases what the nurse believes the patient is saying, such as "It sounds as though you don't understand the importance of exercise." The goals of reflective listening are to assist the patient to state goals for change and to validate the patient's feelings and ideas.

31. C: The biggest obstacle to long-term management of cardiovascular disease is non-adherence to treatment regimens. Compliance with treatment varies according to duration, with adherence decreasing fairly markedly during the first year and then gradually continuing to decrease over time. Patients are resistive to lifestyle changes, especially with long-term adherence to smoking cessation, weight reduction, and exercise programs. Up to 10% of patients do not even fill prescriptions for medications, and many patients take a lesser dosage than prescribed or stop taking medications.

32. C: The primary purpose of the Patient Learning Needs Scale (PLNS) is to plan education for discharge. The PLNS is a self-administered test with 50 questions, such as "What are possible side effects of treatments?" The patient scores each question according to its importance:

1. Not important
2. Slightly important
3. Moderately important
4. Very important
5. Extremely important

The individual scores help to provide information about specific training needs, while the overall score provides information about the patient's health literacy and confidence in providing self-care after discharge.

33. D: While developmental stages have traditionally been viewed as a mechanism of chronology, based on a patient's age and the passage of time, there are other influences that affect development:

- Normative age-graded: factors that are similar to those of the approximate age, such as puberty and menopause
- Normative history-graded: factors that are common to a particular cohort of people, such as the September 11, 2001 terrorist attack, the Korean Conflict, the Vietnam War, and the computer age
- Normative life events: factors that cause a change in life, such as birth of children, serious injury, and divorce

34. B: For percutaneous transluminal coronary angioplasty (PTCA) to be considered successful, residual stenosis after balloon inflation should be less than 30%. PTCA is most effective for discrete concentric lesions of less than 10 mm, and treatment is more successful if the patient has experienced angina for less than a year because the lesions are less calcified and easier to compress. Stenting, atherectomy, and laser angioplasty may be done to prevent closure of the artery.

35. D: Considering barriers to learning, changes in fluid intelligence associated with aging may result in altered perception of time. This may cause people to put off learning or dealing with issues, believing that they have plenty of time. Other barriers include slow processing time, slower reaction time, and persistence of stimulus (confusing a new word/information with a previous one). Older adults also tend to have decreased short-term memory and increased test anxiety.

36. A: The goal of older adults most likely to increase their motivation to learn is independence. Older adults especially want to maintain independence so that they can avoid being a burden to others and will engage in health teaching that increases their chance of remaining independent. Older adults also want to gain approval and social acceptability from others. Personal resources vary widely among older adults, and coping mechanisms may be positive or negative.

37. D: In order to compensate for patients' hearing losses, teaching strategies may include speaking slowly (≤140 words per minute) and in a low-pitched tone, as higher pitched sounds are harder to hear. The nurse should avoid shouting, which distorts sounds. The nurse should also avoid exaggerated lip movements, as it disrupts lip reading. If patients use hearing aids, the nurse should make sure they have batteries and are turned on and properly adjusted.

38. C: When assessing the ankle-brachial index, the Doppler wand should be held at a 45° angle to the skin. The cardiac/vascular nurse should palpate the brachial pulse, apply conductive gel, and obtain the systolic reading with the Doppler wand. For the ankle readings, the nurse should repeat the procedure for both the dorsalis pedis pulse and the posterior tibial pulse, using the highest ankle reading for the calculations (Ankle reading/brachial reading = AB index), which are done separately for each side.

39. B: The six-minute walk test is generally done over a distance of 30 meters, with the starting and stopping points clearly marked. Patients are usually advised to walk as far as possible at their usual pace with whatever walking aids they normally utilize. If encouragement is given, it should be given at regularly spaced intervals (every 30 seconds, every minute) and documented. Patients are often encouraged to do at least two practice walks prior to actual measurement of time and distance.

40. A: If, during the clinical interview, a patient states she is allergic to a medication, the initial response of the cardiac/vascular nurse should be to ask what type of reaction the patient had. In many cases, patients may have experienced an adverse reaction rather than an allergic response, which may be far more serious, but both allergic reactions and adverse reactions should be documented so that clinicians are aware to avoid prescribing the medications.

41. B: According to ACC/AHA guidelines, if a patient is admitted with angina, and the ECG indicates an ST-segment myocardial infarction (STEMI), the next step should be reperfusion therapy, such as thrombolysis or angioplasty. The ECG findings (ST-segment elevation, T-wave inversion, pathologic Q waves) are considered diagnostic in the presence of ischemic pain. Waiting for cardiac markers may result in further cardiac damage and may put the patient outside of the window of time for thrombolysis.

42. B: If a patient's oxygen saturation per pulse oximeter has been stable at 95–96% but suddenly drops to 85% even though the patient does not appear to be in distress, the cardiac/vascular nurse should check and reposition the pulse oximeter before taking further action because an actual sudden drop is likely to result in obvious symptoms, such as dyspnea and tachycardia. Pulse oximeters often become loose or dislodged because of patient activity.

43. C: When using the FICA (faith and belief – importance and influence – community – address in care) rubric for a spiritual assessment of a patient, "community" refers to the religious or support groups that a patient is associated with. This may include a church, temple, synagogue, or mosque or a group of like-minded individuals who provide emotional and spiritual support to each other.

One should not assume that a patient who claims no religious beliefs or affiliations lacks spirituality or a belief in spirituality.

44. D: If a patient reports that he experienced an episode of severe chest pain seven days previously and has had recurrent chest pain, dyspnea, and weakness since that time, the most appropriate cardiac marker to determine if the patient experienced a myocardial infarction is probably troponin T. Myoglobin usually returns to normal levels within 24 hours, CK-MB within 48 hours, troponin I within a week, and troponin T within 12 days, so troponin T would still show an elevation after a week.

45. A: A normal value for troponin I in an adult (over age 18) is under 0.04 ng/mL. Troponin I is the most accurate cardiac marker because it is specific to injury of the myocardium. Troponin I levels increase within 3–6 hours and peak in 14–20 hours, returning to normal within a week. In many cases, the troponin I level alone is adequate to diagnose cardiac injury, although other markers, such as CK-MB, are often done as well.

46. C: B-type natriuretic peptide (BNP) level of 375 pg/mL is consistent with moderate heart failure, requiring light limitation of physical activity. Normal levels should be less than 100 pg/mL, with higher levels indicative of heart failure. The higher the level, the more severe the degree of heart failure. At 250 pg/mL, heart failure is mild but does not require limitation of activities. At 650 pg/mL, heart failure is moderate to severe with marked limitations of activities. At 800 pg/mL, heart failure is severe, and the patient has no tolerance for activities.

47. A: In an ECG tracing, the QRS complex represents ventricular depolarization, which is the wave of conduction moving across the ventricles. The P wave indicates the depolarization wave initiated by the SA node and followed by the QRS complex, with the Q wave showing a downward deflection and the R wave an upward deflection. The T wave, which immediately follows the QRS complex, represents repolarization, reverting to a state of readiness for the next wave of conduction.

48. C: If, when monitoring cardiac telemetry, the cardiac/vascular nurse notes a prominent U wave, this may represent electrolyte imbalance, particularly severe hypokalemia. In some cases, U waves may be a normal variation, although the cause is not clear. Normal U waves are less than 25% the height of T waves, with amplitude of 1–2 mm, while abnormal (prominent) U waves are more than 25% the height of T waves, with amplitude of more than 1–2 mm.

49. B: If a patient complains of angina, the cardiac/vascular nurse recognizes that this usually means that one or more coronary arteries are occluded by at least 70% (usually resulting from atherosclerosis), causing myocardial ischemia because oxygen supply is insufficient for demand. Stable angina tends to be predictable in the sense that it is precipitated by a certain degree of activity and responds to cessation of the activity or treatment with a vasodilator, such as nitroglycerine.

50. D: According to the Venous Thromboembolism Risk Factor Assessment, the factor that poses the greatest risk is a hip fracture within the previous month. Other high-risk factors include elective arthroplasty of the lower extremity and pelvis or leg fracture, stroke, multiple traumas, and acute spinal cord injury with paralysis within the previous month as well as major surgery of over three hours duration. The assessment assigns scores ranging from one to five points to different factors, with the total score used to determine overall risk and need for prophylaxis.

51. B: While a medical translator is preferable to a family member if one is available, especially for history and physical exam, the NIH stroke scale should not be delayed if a family member is able to translate because the instructions for the scale are fairly simple. The patient may not be able to complete the reading portion of the test, but the cardiac/vascular nurse can ask the family member to speak the translated sentences and ask the patient to repeat them because the purpose is to evaluate the quality of speech rather than the ability to read.

52. A: If the cardiac/vascular nurse notes slight edema of the right foot and ankle and the patient complains of pain on palpation in the calf area with dorsiflexion of the foot, the nurse should suspect deep vein thrombosis (DVT) in the calf veins. DVT increases the risk of pulmonary embolism as well as stroke and myocardial infarction, so rapid identification and treatment is critical. The classic triad (Virchow) of symptoms associated with DVT includes (1) blood stasis, (2) increased coagulability, and (3) injury to the vessel wall.

53. C: The complementary/alternative therapy that should generally be avoided in patients with cardiovascular disease is St. John's wort because it reacts negatively with many drugs used in the treatment of cardiovascular disease, such as warfarin, clopidogrel, digoxin, lovastatin, and simvastatin. St. John's wort is an herbal preparation and is used primarily to reduce mild to moderate depression and anxiety. Patients undergoing anesthesia should withhold St. John's wort for at least 14 days prior to surgery, as the combination of the drug and anesthetic may cause cardiac abnormalities.

54. D: When stratifying patients who are to undergo exercise for cardiac rehabilitation according to risk of cardiac events, a rest ejection fraction under 40% would pose the highest degree of risk:

- Low risk: rest ejection fraction 50% or higher, functional capacity 7 METS or higher, normal hemodynamics and absence of angina, ventricular arrhythmias, CHF, or other serious symptoms
- Intermediate risk: angina with activity greater than 7 METS, functional capacity less than 5 METS, rest ejection fraction 40–49%, exercise-induced ST-segment depression less than 2 mm from baseline
- High risk: rest ejection fraction less than 40%, angina with activity less than 5 METS, exercise-induced ST-segment depression at least 2 mm from baseline, complex ventricular arrhythmias and/or abnormal hemodynamics during exercise testing

55. B: If, when teaching a patient how to use a Holter monitor, the patient repeatedly says, "Can I see that?" and "Show me...", this suggests that the best teaching aids may be pictures and diagrams because the questions are focused on visual-spatial aspects of learning rather than factual information delivered in language format. Patients who ask such questions as "Can you explain that again?" may prefer written materials so that they can read instructions.

56. A: If a patient with heart failure has a nursing diagnosis of decreased cardiac output, an appropriate Nursing Outcome Classification (NOC) for this diagnosis is cardiac pump effectiveness. Appropriate Nursing Intervention Classifications (NICs) for this diagnosis include cardiac care, hemodynamic regulation, and teaching: disease process. The common expected outcomes are that the patient's vital signs will remain within normal limits, with regular cardiac rhythm and equal peripheral pulses, with skin warm and dry, and with lungs clear bilaterally.

57. D: According to the ACCF/AHA Guideline for the Management of Heart Failure, patients at Stage A of risk for heart failure because of hypertension and/or diabetes mellitus but without structural heart disease or heart failure symptoms should be treated with ACEIs or ARBs as well as statins as appropriate. At risk patients at Stage B exhibit signs of structural heart disease but no signs of heart failure. Stage B may include patients with previous MI and left ventricular remodeling with LVH and low ejection fraction or asymptomatic valve disease. ACEIs, ARBs, and beta-blockers as well as revascularization procedures may be indicated.

58. B: Heart failure is defined according to ejection fraction:

- EF of ≤40% indicates heart failure with reduced ejection fraction.
- EF of 41–49% indicates heart failure with borderline ejection fraction.
- EF of 50–70% indicates a normal ejection fraction.
- EF of >75% may indicate hypertrophic cardiomyopathy.

59. A: When a patient is at rest, the percentage of the total blood volume that is generally contained in the heart and pulmonary bed is 15–25%. The majority of the blood volume, 60–80%, is contained in the systemic veins, with a quarter to a half of this volume in small veins less than 1 mm in diameter. About 25% of the total blood volume is in the splanchnic circulation. About 10% of the total blood volume is in the aorta and systemic arteries, and 5% is in capillaries.

60. B: Hypoxia occurs when oxygen at the tissue level is inadequate for body needs. Hypoxia is classified according to the cause:

- Ischemic hypoxia: Hypoxia is caused by decreased blood flow to the tissues.
- Anemic hypoxia: PO_2 is normal but the hemoglobin level and thus oxygen-carrying capacity is reduced.
- Hypoxic hypoxia: PO_2 level is decreased and inadequate.
- Histotoxic hypoxia: Oxygen delivery to the tissue is normal, but the cells are unable to utilize the oxygen or produce ATP.

61. C: A coronary atherosclerotic lesion that is 25 mm in length with angulated segments of more than 90° is classified according to ACC/AHA guidelines as Class C, putting the patient at high risk for complications after reperfusion interventions, such as PCI, and for recurrent symptoms. Class A lesions (low risk) are less than 10 mm in length with non-angulated segment of less than 45°. Class B lesions (moderate risk) are 10–20 mm in length with moderately angulated segment of 45–90°. There is no Class D.

62. A: Warfarin is an antagonist of vitamin K. Warfarin inhibits the vitamin K-dependent activation of clotting factors II, VII, IX, and X, so the anticoagulation effects are neutralized by the oral or parenteral administration of vitamin K. Patients should be advised to look for signs of bleeding, such as ecchymosis, melena, hematuria, and purple-toe syndrome (purplish discoloration of toes that may occur 3–10 weeks or later after initiation of treatment), as severe bleeding can occur, especially during initial administration and/or with high doses.

63. D: If a patient taking a cardiac glycoside (digoxin) is also to take a calcium channel blocker (verapamil), the dosage of the cardiac glycoside should be decreased by 50% because the CCB decreases the clearance of the cardiac glycoside, so continuing at the same dose may result in digoxin toxicity. Cardiac glycosides must be taken with care with other cardiovascular medications. For example, combining cardiac glycosides with loop or thiazide diuretics may cause hypokalemia. Additionally, both CCBs and beta-blockers may enhance the bradycardic effects of the cardiac glycoside.

64. A: Digoxin should be withheld for a minimum of 48 hours before cardioversion. Anticoagulation, usually with warfarin (Coumadin), is prescribed at least three weeks before cardioversion to prevent emboli. Sometimes drug therapy is used in conjunction with cardioversion: for example, antiarrhythmics (Cardizem, Cordarone) may be given before the procedure to slow the heart rate. Insulin should not be withheld for 48 hours, but the patient must fast before cardioversion and may be asked to delay the insulin injection on the morning of the procedure.

65. C: If a patient has undergone thrombolysis per accelerated infusion of alteplase 100 mg (maximum dose) for an acute myocardial infarction and shows 20% reduction in ST elevation after 90 minutes, the cardiac/vascular nurse anticipates angiography and rescue PCI because ST elevation should decrease by at least 50% within this timeframe. Fibrinolytic therapy is often administered instead of PCI if PCI is not available at the hospital or within an acceptable period of time, so arrangements should be made to transfer the patient to another facility if necessary.

66. D: If a patient complains loudly about her physician and states that the physician is incompetent, the best response is: "You're concerned that you are not getting better." This reflects the real meaning patients often have behind criticism of their healthcare providers and moves the focus from the physician back to the patient in order to allow the patient to express real concerns. The cardiac/vascular nurse should avoid advice statements ("You should...") or direct or implied threatening statements ("Do you want another physician?").

67. C: If the cardiac/vascular nurse is providing treatment to an older Japanese female patient but the patient does not make eye contact and responds very quietly, this behavior probably represents respect for the nurse. Avoiding eye contact as a sign of respect is very common among Asian cultures as is speaking in a low tone of voice. Asian patients may expect the nurse to be an authority and may follow directions without question and may not feel comfortable saying they do not understand.

68. C: For a patient about to be discharged after implantation of a pacemaker, the role of the faith community nurse is primarily to assess patient's needs and make referrals, ensuring that the patient is able to access community services and spiritual guidance. The faith community nurse may be employed by one or more churches or may act as a volunteer, but the nurse is rarely expected to provide actual physical nursing care of the patient.

69. B: An appropriate role of the home health nurse for a patient being discharged from an acute care hospital after a myocardial infarction with PCI (angioplasty) is to monitor vital signs and treatment adherence. While the home health nurse may administer IV medications, the nurse does not generally administer daily oral medications, although the nurse may educate the patient about the medications and help set up weekly dosage dispensers if necessary. The nurse does not transport the patient or provide assistance in hiring a housekeeper.

70. D: If the cardiac/vascular nurse is participating in a health fair at the local shopping mall, offering a service, such as a BP check, is the most appropriate activity to attract visitors to the nurse's booth because people, by nature, like to receive something of value in return for attention. Once a person stops at the booth for the BP check (a valuable screening for hypertension), the nurse can provide brochures and information about follow-up for people with elevated BP.

71. A: According to the ACC/AHA Guideline on the Assessment of Cardiovascular Risk, race- and gender-specific Pooled Cohort Equations should be used to predict 10-year risk for a first hard atherosclerotic cardiovascular disease (ASCVD) event for all non-Hispanic African Americans and non-Hispanic whites, ages 40–79. The ACC/AHA Guideline notes that this tool may overestimate or underestimate this risk for the Hispanic population. Risk factors should be assessed for all adults (ages 20–79) who are free of ASCVD every 4–6 years, and the 10-year risk should be estimated in those ages 40–70 every 4–6 years.

72. A: According to ACC/AHA guidelines, exercise electrography is recommended for cardiovascular screening only for symptomatic adults, but no value is found for its use for routine screening for asymptomatic adults with low risk factors, and false positives often lead to costly and unnecessary invasive tests. Risk factors include age over 45, male gender, and lifestyle habits (smoking). Exercise electrography is not recommended for those whose risk assessment is equal to or less than 10%.

73. B: When conducting a sleep assessment for a patient with heart failure, the cardiac/vascular nurse recognizes that the two cardinal signs of sleep apnea are snoring and daytime sleepiness. With obstructive sleep apnea, patients may stop breathing for periods lasting 10 seconds or longer. Obstructive sleep apnea occurs when a collapsed upper airway blocks to flow of air despite effort to breathe, resulting in brief arousal and intake of breath. Obstructive sleep apnea is most common in overweight middle-aged males and post-menopausal females.

74. D: If, when conducting an assessment of a patient's retina, the cardiac/vascular nurse notes a silver wire artery, this usually indicates hypertension. With high blood pressure, the walls of retinal arteries begin to thicken, and the lumens narrow, resulting in a narrow column of blood and narrowed light reflex so that the artery is increasingly opaque. If the blood column is so narrow that the blood cannot be observed, this is referred to as a silver wire artery because it is completely opaque.

75. C: If the abdominojugular reflux (AKA hepatojugular reflux) shows a rise in the jugular venous pressure of 4 cm (at least 3 cm) throughout pressure application, this indicates right ventricular failure and may also be observed with constrictive pericarditis, cardiac tamponade, and tricuspid regurgitation. Abdominojugular reflux is assessed by applying firm pressure (30–40 mmHg) to the periumbilical area for 30–60 seconds while observing the jugular venous pressure.

76. A: When measuring and documenting paradoxical blood pressure, the first documented systolic sound is that heard on expiration. The patient should be advised to lie quietly and breathe normally. The air in the cuff must be released very slowly, and some reinflation may be necessary to isolate sounds. After the initial recording of the systolic sound on expiration, the next recording is the point where sound is heard both on inspiration and expiration. The difference between the two recordings (the paradox) should be less than 10 mm.

77. A: A summation gallop can be heard on auscultation of the heart in the presence of cardiac failure with tachycardia. If cardiac failure is severe with both systolic and diastolic dysfunction, four distinct heart sounds can often be heard (S1, S2, S3, and S4); however, if the heartbeat is rapid, as with tachycardia, then the S3 and S4 sounds tend to fuse together into one loud sound, the summation gallop.

78. A: The reference range for the cardiac marker CK-MB is 0–5%. CK-MB is more specific to myocardial infarction than other cardiac injury, such as trauma or cardiac catheterization. CK-MB levels increase within 4–6 hours of an MI and peak at 12–24 hours, returning to normal values within 3–4 days. While specific to the myocardium, CK-MB is less specific than troponin I, although both tests are frequently ordered.

79. C: If the echocardiogram indicates increased left ventricular intracavity dimension and decreased ventricular wall movements, these findings are consistent with dilated cardiomyopathy (AKA congestive or ischemic cardiomyopathy). Because the myocardial muscle fibers are damaged,

LV contractility decreases, resulting in decreased cardiac output, ejection fraction, and stroke volume. All chambers of the heart begin to dilate, resulting in a heart that is globular-shaped and enlarged. Dilated cardiomyopathy is most common in males over 55, and prognosis is poor.

80. C: The diagnostic procedure that is most indicated for suspected aortic dissection in a stable patient is MRI, as it provides better visualization of the intravascular and extravascular spaces as well as the walls of the aorta, compared to CT, transthoracic echocardiogram, or x-ray. MRI may also be used to diagnose or monitor complex congenital heart disease, arrhythmogenic right ventricular dysplasia (ARVD), and intracardiac or paracardiac lesions. MRI does not require use of radiation and allows for capture of 2-D and 3-D images.

81. D: When estimating the heart rate from an ECG strip, the cardiac/vascular nurse should begin by counting the number of R-R intervals in a 6-second strip and multiplying that number by 10 (because 10 six-second strips occur in a one-minute tracing). One minute also has 300 large boxes on the graph, so another method (if the pulse is regular) is to count the number of large boxes between two R waves and divide 300 by that number or count the number of small boxes between two R waves and divide that number into 1500.

82. B: Lack of social/family support would make a patient ineligible for a left ventricular assist device (LVAD) because patients must adhere to a strict medical regimen and must be able to identify a person who can remain with the patient constantly for the first weeks after discharge from the hospital, who can attend training sessions, and who can ensure the patient has transportation to appointments. The three primary reasons for insertion of a LVAD are (1) bridge to transplant, (2), bridge to recovery, and (3), destination therapy for those ineligible for transplant.

83. A: If a patient is to be discharged after a pacemaker is implanted in the chest, the patient should be advised to avoid the distributor of a gas-operated engine (while the engine is running). Patients need not avoid microwave ovens or electric hand tools and may walk through anti-theft security gates (or airport security) but should keep moving and avoid standing in the security gates for a prolonged period of time. If a detection wand is used to scan the patient, the patient should advise the examiner to avoid scanning the pacemaker.

84. B: If a patient is wearing a LifeVest and hears the device sound an alarm but feels all right, the patient should press buttons to stop the shock sequence, as there is a delay between the alarm and the shock (usually of about 25 seconds). If the LifeVest is sending false alarms, then the patient should notify the physician or reposition the LifeVest. The LifeVest activates when the continuous monitor detects ventricular fibrillation or ventricular tachycardia.

85. D: When teaching a patient to manage wound care prior to discharge following CABG, the best method to ensure that the patient understands the procedure is to utilize teach-back, which includes teaching the patient and then asking the patient to demonstrate and explain the procedure. Teach-back helps to reinforce the teaching by facilitating retention and helps the nurse identify areas that may need more instruction or clarification. One method of teach-back is to say, "Tell me what you will do when you change your dressing at home."

86. D: Under Healthy People 2030, the objective is to decrease stroke-related deaths from 37.1 per 100,000 in 2018, to 33.4 per 100,000 by 2030. Recommended interventions to meet this objective include monitoring and managing blood pressure, diet, and exercise in addition to increasing awareness of the symptoms and what to do if a stroke is suspected.

87. C: While volunteer programs (such as Friendly Visitor Program) vary widely, most volunteers are not licensed or bonded and do not provide direct patient care or other services. They may do light tasks, such as deliver meals, pick up the mail, or read to a patient, but their primary responsibility is usually to provide social interaction and companionship for homebound patients. They may visit the patient in the home as well as maintain contact through the Internet or telephone.

88. A: The purpose of paratransit services, mandated by the ADA for patients who qualify as disabled, is to provide transportation from a requested address to a destination, such as from home to a doctor's office or adult daycare program and then back home again. Patients may usually request service with 24-hour notice and may set up routine services for regular appointments or scheduled programs. Programs usually require physician authorization and payment for rides.

89. A: If a patient with coronary artery disease wants to quit smoking but is unable to attend smoking cessation classes because of health problems and lack of transportation, the best resource that the cardiac/vascular nurse can provide is probably 1-800-QUIT-NOW, which is the national helpline connected to helplines in each state. The helplines are staffed with counselors who will help the patient work out an individualized plan and refer the patient to a variety of other services, including social support message boards.

90. D: In order to participate in a pharmaceutical assistance program, the patient must apply directly to the manufacturer. The patient may begin at Medicare.gov, which has links to manufacturers. The patient searches by medication name and then clicks on a link that gives information, including the name of the company, the drug program, the eligibility criteria, the benefits and assistance, and contact information. Programs vary widely but are need-based and may have income/insurance restrictions.

91. A: If a patient with no family wants to ensure that her advance directive is respected, the cardiac/vascular nurse should recommend that the patient give copies to all her physicians and healthcare providers. If the patient has close friends, then these people should also have a copy. Because advance directives are not legally binding in most states, and physicians often defer to family members, the patient with no family should convey her wishes to as many healthcare providers as she can, being very clear about her wishes.

92. D: The primary purpose for using the SBAR (situation-background-assessment-recommendation) method for hand-off procedures is to promote patient safety by ensuring that all pertinent information is conveyed during hand-off. Organizations utilizing SBAR have guidelines advising staff exactly what should be covered in each element and a worksheet the providers can utilize to organize information. The SBAR method was originally intended for communication between a nurse and physician, but the method has been extended to other healthcare professionals.

93. A: If a patient has developed a life-threatening arrhythmia and the cardiac/vascular nurse notifies the physician on call but, when the physician arrives, the nurse notes that the physician smells of alcohol and has slurred speech, the nurse should immediately notify a supervisor. As an advocate for the patient and from an ethical standpoint, the cardiac/vascular cannot allow an impaired clinician to care for the patient, even if this means confronting the physician if there is no other recourse.

94. B: If a patient confides to the cardiac/vascular nurse that the antihypertensive medication he has been taking has resulted in increasing impotence, so he has decreased the dosage and frequency, the best response is: "You need to talk to the physician about changing the medication or dosage." The cardiac/vascular nurse should assure the patient that the physician may be able to help him if the patient talks honestly with the physician and should stress the risks involved in changing the dosage or frequency of the medication.

95. D: The cardiac/vascular nurse should take responsibility for an improper delegation. Of the five rights of delegation—right task, right circumstance, right person, right direction/communication, and right supervision/evaluation—the nurse violated at least the last three rights. The nurse did not determine if the UAP was adequately trained, so the wrong person was delegated. The nurse did not communicate clearly about the need to know how to do the procedure and did not adequately supervise to ensure that the procedure was done correctly.

96. D: If the cardiac/vascular nurse notes that a patient seems angry and upset after the doctor has left, a response that exemplifies therapeutic communication is: "Is there anything you'd like to talk about." This is an open-ended question that encourages a patient to share without probing ("Why are you so upset?"). The nurse should not ask for explanations about behavior or feelings that are unrelated to care, as this is intrusive. The nurse should also avoid meaningless clichés ("Try not to worry…") and should avoid giving advice ("You should…").

97. B: In order to successfully manage conflict in the workplace, the management must first recognize the existence of conflict and consider the impact it has on work dynamics. Open communication and showing respect to all parties of a conflict are important considerations. All members of an organization must be educated about conflict resolution and understand their individual roles in ensuring that conflict is managed effectively and should understand that they will be held accountable for utilizing the process in place.

98. D: A patient with aortic stenosis eligible for transcatheter aortic valve replacement (TAVR) must not be a candidate for open-chest surgery, as the procedure is not yet approved for those patients. The femoral approach (similar to angioplasty) is the most common, with a bovine valve and metal stent positioned inside the existing valve per the catheter. Once in proper position, the balloon is inflated, securing the valve and stent, and then the catheter is removed.

99. A: If an 18-year-old Jehovah's Witness patient begins to hemorrhage following open-heart surgery and signs consent for blood transfusions, the nurse should administer the blood transfusion because the patient's parents have no legal standing since the patient is legally an adult and can make all decisions about his own healthcare. The nurse should explain this to the parents without getting into an argument. Jehovah Witnesses are prohibited by their religion from accepting whole blood or its components but may receive fractions, such as clotting factors, from RBCs, WBCs, platelets, and plasma.

100. C: A criterion for endovascular thoracic aortic aneurysm repair is an aneurysm in the descending thoracic aorta that is at least double the size of the adjacent aorta (greater than 5 cm in diameter). Also, there must be adequate normal aorta on either side so that the stent graft can properly adhere. Diseases affecting the connective tissue, such as Marfan disease, are contraindications because the tissue may not remain stable. Patients must receive annual CT scans to check for endoleaks or other complications after surgery.

101. A: Elective cardioversion is synchronized with the ECG, and the current is delivered during the QRS complex (ventricular depolarization) in order to prevent VT or VF. Patients generally receive anticoagulants (such as warfarin) for three weeks prior to cardioversion to prevent emboli. Digoxin should be withheld for three days before the procedure. The patient usually receives sedation or anesthesia for cardioversion. In some cases, antiarrhythmics, such as diltiazem, may be administered prior to the procedure as well.

102. D: According to the ACC/AHA Focused Update of the Guideline for the Management of Patients with Peripheral Artery Disease, ASA 75 mg to 325 mg or clopidogrel 75 mg is recommended to reduce risk of MI, stroke, or vascular death in patients with atherosclerotic lower extremity peripheral arterial disease. Warfarin and other anticoagulants are not recommended. For severe cases, such as those with critical limb ischemia, a combination of clopidogrel and ASA may be considered.

103. A: According to the Eighth Report of the Joint National Committee on Prevention, Detection, Evaluation, and Treatment of High Blood Pressure, when lifestyle changes alone do not control blood pressure, the first drug of choice should be one of the following: thiazide diuretic, angiotensin receptor blocker, ACE inhibitor, or calcium channel blocker alone, or in combination, based on the patient's race and comorbidities. Should this medication addition not work, the JNC 8 recommends adding a second of those initial drugs. Should this combination of medications not work, only then would a beta-blocker be recommended to treat hypertension.

104. B: To ensure correct fit of a blood pressure cuff and correct readings, the cuff bladder should encircle at least 80% of the arm. Cuff sizes are:

- Small adult: 10 cm width/24 cm length for arm circumference of 22–26 cm
- Adult: 13 cm width/30 cm length for arm circumference of 27–34 cm
- Large adult: 16 cm width/38 cm length for arm circumference of 35–44 cm
- Extra-large adult/Thigh: 20 cm width/42 cm length for arm/thigh circumference of 45–52 cm

105. D: If a patient has high blood pressure readings during visits with clinicians but reports lower blood pressure readings at home, the best solution is to conduct ambulatory blood pressure monitoring (ABPM) while the patient goes about normal activities. Patients often become tense when examined by a clinician and may exhibit "white coat" hypertension. A 24-hour BP recording provides multiple values and can show how the BP varies throughout the day and night, and the average can help predict risk of cardiovascular event.

106. B: According to the Eighth Report of the Joint National Committee on Prevention, Detection, Evaluation, and Treatment of High Blood Pressure, 10 ounces of wine per day is acceptable for a male patient (two 5-ounce glasses). Male patients should imbibe no more than 1 ounce of ethanol daily, and female patients should imbibe no more than 0.5 ounces.

	Male	**Female**
Beer	24 ounces	12 ounces
Wine	10 ounces	5 ounces
80-proof whiskey	3 ounces	1.5 ounces

107. A: Thiazide diuretics are recommended as the preferred initial antihypertensive agent for preventing complications of hypertension. Thiazide diuretics, such as chlorothiazide, chlorthalidone, hydrochlorothiazide, and indapamide, are well tolerated and have few adverse effects compared to other antihypertensives. Studies show that patients treated with calcium channel blockers or ACE inhibitors are at higher risk for developing heart failure than those treated with thiazide diuretics. However, higher thiazide doses may increase risk of gout because of increased uric acid levels.

108. B: If a Middle Eastern patient admitted for heart failure is found to have a number of annular ecchymotic regions up and down the back with some evidence of hematoma and small lacerations, the most likely reason is wet cupping, a traditional healing practice. With wet cupping, the skin is lanced and then a heated cup is placed over the area. Suction is created as the air inside the cup cools. This cupping often leaves annular bruising and, if lancing took place, hematomas or small lacerations may be evident.

109. D: If a patient exhibits resistant hypertension, the first thing to evaluate before changing medications is the accuracy of blood pressure readings, ensuring that the cuff size is correct, the BP equipment is properly calibrated, and the reading is done correctly. Ambulatory blood pressure monitoring may be indicated before any changes in medications. Volume overload because of sodium retention or inadequate diuretic therapy should be evaluated. Drugs should be evaluated for adherence, dosage, and interactions, and lifestyle (diet, obesity, smoking, exercise, and alcohol intake) should be examined.

110. B: If a patient who has been hospitalized for a week asks the cardiac/vascular nurse, who lives in the patient's neighborhood, to go by the patient's house and water her plants after work, the nurse should offer to help the patient contact a friend or neighbor. The nurse must use care not to violate professional boundaries of attention, which would include carrying out favors for a patient beyond what is expected. Additionally, if later on the patient believes items are missing from her home, the nurse may be suspected.

111. A: If a cardiac/vascular nurse suspects that a patient is not adhering to lifestyle modifications and is lying about doing so and telephones the patient's brother for information about the patient without telling the patient, this is an example of a Health Insurance Portability and Accountability Act (HIPAA) violation because the nurse does not have reason to believe that the patient would not object and did not ask the patient's permission.

112. D: Because of changing demographics and increased costs of medical care, future medical care will likely place more emphasis on preventive care. Currently, there is a move toward decreasing acute hospitalization and rehospitalization by better management of patient care and by shifting resources to home-based and community-based care. Under CMS guidelines and the Affordable Care Act, more preventive measures, such as vaccinations and routine screenings, are covered by Medicare and insurance policies.

113. C: If a cardiac/vascular nurse conducts literature research and proposes a different approach to patient triage based on evidence-based practices, and the practice improves efficiency and the quality of patient care, the nurse could be best described as a change agent. A change agent is someone in an organization who facilitates change, usually with a positive outcome. While being a change agent is a valuable quality for a leader, one does not have to be a leader to recognize the need for change and to take action.

114. D: According to the diffusion of innovation theory, when innovative change is proposed, the adopter category likely to include the smallest number of individuals is innovators. Categories are:

- Innovators (2.5%): These are excited about trying changes.
- Early adopters (13.5%): These help to bring about acceptance.
- Early majority (34%): These see the advantages of change and cooperate.
- Late majority (34%): These learn from those who have already adopted change but are somewhat skeptical.
- Laggards (16%): These remain resistant to change, regardless of its benefits.

115. A: When promoting change within an organization, the cardiac/vascular nurse should recognize that the primary means by which staff members interpret and understand the dynamics of change is per informal communication with peers. Thus, the nurse who advocates for change should participate in as many discussions as possible and engage those who are the recipients of change because these staff members will translate and edit plans for change and may be responsible for resistance or acceptance.

116. B: The nominal group technique (NGT) may be most useful in resolving conflicts during meetings. With the NGT, conflict is avoided during brainstorming because it is done as a silent process. Members write down their goals or ideas independently without discussion, and then in a round-robin fashion, each person reads what they have written while another person writes the ideas on a flip chart. Only after all ideas are recorded does discussion take place to clarify and evaluate. Then members independently and privately rank the items with the ranking tallied to determine priorities.

117. C: If, in an interdisciplinary team, one member frequently and effusively praises one of the other members, this is an example of a member trying to gain influence over another through ingratiation. Other tactics used to influence others are assertiveness (speaking forcefully without downgrading others' ideas), exchange (something offered for something gained), rationality (providing logical arguments), blocking (deliberately preventing others from getting their way), coalitions (banding together), sanctions (threats), and upward appeal.

118. B: A patient who has a very poor prognosis but appears quite cheerful and talks about her plans for a long vacation in Europe after she leaves the hospital is probably using the defense mechanism of denial in order to avoid the stress of dealing with the reality of her prognosis. Denial is a very common method of coping, and, in fact, may reduce a patient's anxiety, at least in the short term. While the goal of nurse-patient communication is to be honest, forcing people to accept the reality of their situation before they are ready is not appropriate.

119. D: If an illegal Mexican immigrant without insurance is treated in the ED for a myocardial infarction, the best referral on discharge in most states is likely a free clinic, such as RotaCare, which may be able to provide assistance with monitoring and medications. Public health departments do not provide the type of follow-up care and treatment the patient needs, and Medicaid programs are prohibited by federal law from providing services to illegal immigrants. Consulates provide little or no help.

120. A: If a physician has ordered an expensive new drug for a patient who has minimal insurance, and the patient tells the nurse that she cannot pay her child's college tuition and pay the medication costs as well, the cardiac/vascular nurse should first discuss the situation with the physician, who may not be aware of the financial concerns, to determine whether another medication can be substituted. Patients are very often reluctant to discuss financial matters with physicians.

121. D: If a patient has a nursing diagnosis of extracellular fluid volume excess and one of the goals is to prevent specific manifestations of extracellular fluid volume excess, appropriate outcome criteria for this goal include: "Patient maintains normal weight and exhibits no S3, crackles, or peripheral edema." Interventions include teaching the patient about any dietary restrictions (sodium, calories, fluid), daily weight monitoring, and exercise regimens.

122. B: The primary treatment focus for patients with dilated cardiomyopathy is controlling heart failure by improving myocardial contractility and decreasing afterload. Patients may take a variety of medications, including diuretics, nitrates, ACE inhibitors, beta-blockers, antidysrhythmics, and anticoagulants. However, dilated cardiomyopathy does not readily respond to medications, and patients may experience repeated episodes of heart failure. Some patients may receive a ventricular-assist device, especially while awaiting transplant.

123. A: If, when an elderly patient is to be removed from life support, his daughter complains loudly that her father was selfish and brought his illness on himself by refusing to cooperate with his physicians, the daughter's reaction is probably an expression of grief. The five stages of grief include denial, anger, bargaining, depression, and acceptance. Many people, such as this daughter, react with anger, sometimes lashing out at other family members, caregivers, or even, as in this case, the patient.

124. C: If a patient is awaiting surgical intervention for a dissecting aortic aneurysm, prior to surgery, the patient's systolic blood pressure should be maintained at 110–120 mmHg to ensure adequate perfusion of the patient's organs while preventing undue pressure on the dissection. The patient should receive medications to reduce pain and anxiety, as these symptoms may increase the blood pressure. Antihypertensive agents should be administered under close supervision with constant monitoring of ECG recordings and vital signs.

125. D: If an implantable ICD must be turned off for a procedure, the safest method is to carefully follow manufacturer's instructions, which may vary from one manufacturer to another. While it has been common practice to apply a magnet over an ICD to temporarily turn the ICD off, in fact, this procedure does not work for all manufacturers because some ICDs can be programmed to NOT respond to application of a magnet.

126. A: The precaution that is necessary for a patient with an implanted ICD is that cell phones should be more than 6 inches away from the ICD implantation site (encourage patient to use the phone on the opposite side) because the ICD may mistake the cell phone signal for the heartbeat. Scanning with hand-held security detectors should be under 30 seconds. Patients should stand at least 2 feet away from arc welding equipment. Patients are usually advised to avoid driving for one week after implantation or up to 6 months if implantation followed a sudden cardiac arrest/ventricular arrhythmia.

127. B: From the perspective of risk management, the best method to improve patient safety is probably better training for healthcare providers about patient safety as well as instituting a number of practices that will reduce errors, such as notifying patients when prescriptions will expire, providing follow-up for missing tests or appointments, improving communication with patients, instituting measures to prevent falls, reinforcing the need for handwashing, and documenting accurately and in a timely manner.

128. D: If a patient has suspected endocarditis, the diagnostic tests most indicated are blood cultures and echocardiogram. The patient should be treated initially with a broad-spectrum antibiotic and changed to the most appropriate antibiotic based on results of cultures and sensitivities. The patient should be monitored for conduction defects. If valvular regurgitation is noted, then agents to reduce afterload are indicated. Blood cultures should be repeated after three days of antibiotic therapy.

129. C: The Unna boot with gauze impregnated with zinc oxide, glycerine, or gelatin must always be applied from the toes up toward the knee (distally to proximally), with the wrapping started beneath the patient's first metatarsal. The wrapping is done semi-horizontally at an angle to prevent undue compression, with each circle overlapping the previous by about 50%. Two to three layers of impregnated gauze may be applied and then covered with an ACE bandage or stretch bandage.

130. B: After application of a radial pressure device, if the cardiac/vascular nurse notes a small amount of blood oozing from the puncture site, the next step is to slowly increase the pressure until the bleeding stops. It's important to avoid tightening the device excessively because this can impair circulation. The patient should not be left unattended while the pressure device is in place, and circulation in the hand should be carefully monitored.

131. A: The primary cause of mitral stenosis in patients is rheumatic fever, which can result in fibrinous thickening of the leaflets, fusion of the chordae, and calcification, causing a funnel-shaped valve with the orifice reduced in size from the normal range of 4–6 cm to the point that the left atrium cannot adequately empty and the pressure buildup results in dilation and left atrial hypertrophy. The pressure in the left atrium results in pulmonary hypertension, with the patient experiencing left-sided heart failure without dysfunction of the left ventricle. Increased pulmonary pressure ultimately results in right-sided heart failure as well.

132. D: Following ethanol alcohol septal ablation in a patient with hypertrophic cardiomyopathy, the patient must be carefully monitored for right bundle branch block as well as complete heart block and ventricular tachycardia. Ethanol alcohol septal ablation may result in scar formation, so it is a second line procedure, with septal myomectomy the preferred surgical procedure. During ethanol alcohol septal ablation, a temporary pacemaker is utilized because of the potential for heart block, and up to about 25% or more of patients undergoing the procedure require permanent pacemakers.

133. A: According to the ACCP Antithrombotic Therapy and Prevention of Thrombosis guideline, a patient with suspected recurrent lower extremity DVT should have compression ultrasound as the initial diagnostic procedure. Compression ultrasound can be done at bedside within a few minutes. The procedure is done after applying gel to the leg, probe, or both, with the probe pressed into the vein to completely collapse the vein and partially collapse the artery and then released, repeating this procedure down the length of the veins and arteries.

134. D: Under the Americans with Disabilities Act (ADA), public transportation authorities are required to provide access for people with disabilities, and the patient should qualify because of the severe myocardial infarction. In accordance with ADA regulations, unless it causes undue burden, transportation authorities are required to provide paratransit services, and these services are available in most larger towns and cities. Paratransit services pick up patients at requested addresses and drop them off at their destinations.

135. C: The congenital heart disease that poses a low risk to the pregnant patient is a small, unrepaired ventricular septal defect. Other low risk defects include isolated pulmonic stenosis, tricuspid aortic valve (functionally normal), and postoperative repair of atrial septal defect, ventricular septal defect, tetralogy of Fallot, and patent ductus arteriosus with no residual defect. Intermediate risk occurs with unrepaired aortic value disease, coarctation of aorta, Ebstein anomaly, and congenital corrected transposition of great arteries as well as repairs with residual problems. High risk occurs with cyanotic congenital heart disease, increased pulmonary vascular resistance, and heart failure (NYHA III and IV).

136. C: If a Spanish-speaking Hispanic male patient being monitored in an outpatient clinic has set appointment times but rarely arrives at the scheduled time, sometimes coming early but often arriving one to two hours late, the most likely reason is a cultural perception of time that is more fluid than is common in American culture. Sometimes, compliance will be better if the appointment is associated with some marker, such as asking the patient to come immediately before lunch (being sure to ascertain mealtimes).

137. D: African Americans respond less effectively to ACE inhibitors, ARBs, and beta-blockers than do those in other ethnic groups, although African Americans respond slightly better than others to diuretics and respond effectively to calcium channel blockers. African Americans have the highest rates of hypertension of any ethnic group and develop it at a younger age than others. African American females have higher rates than African American males. Both African Americans and Caucasians living in the Southern part of the United States have higher rates than those living in other parts of the country.

138. C: If a patient is admitted to the cardiac care unit in hypertensive crisis with BP of 240/140 and is started on IV sodium nitroprusside, the initial treatment goal should be to reduce BP by 25% within 60 minutes, with a goal of lowering the BP to 160/100–110 over the next 2–6 hours and then gradually reducing the BP further over 24–48 hours. Lowering the BP too rapidly may result in a stroke. Patients with dissecting aortic aneurysm or acute ischemic stroke may require faster reduction in BP in preparation for other interventions.

139. B: If, when assisting a patient with lifestyle management, the cardiac/vascular nurse notes that the patient's BMI is 31 kg/m^2 and her waist measurement is 39 inches, these findings would classify the patient as obese. A waist measurement of at least 40 inches for a male and at least 35 inches for a female is considered obese. BMI categories are as follows:

- 18.5–24.9 = normal
- 25–29.9 = overweight
- 30–34.9 = obese
- 35–39.9 = severely obese
- 40 + = morbidly obese

140. A: When a patient is using the Borg Rating of Perceived Exertion (RPE) Scale (6 to 20) to rate the amount of effort an activity requires, walking slowly for a few minutes without problems is usually quantified as 9 on the scale. Activities that require no exertion are scored as 6; extremely light activities as 7; very light activities (such as walking by a healthy person) as 9; light activities as 11; somewhat difficult activities as 13; difficult activities as 15; very difficult activities as 17; extremely difficult activities as 19; and maximal exertion activities as 20.

141. D: Isotonic exercises and activities, such as walking, jogging, swimming, and riding a bicycle, are dynamic and involve rhythmic changes in the length of muscles and joint movement with low muscle tension, putting a relatively safe, steady load on the cardiopulmonary system and improving circulation. On the other hand, isometric exercises or activities, such as lifting, carrying, and pushing, are static and increase muscle tension and heart rate, so isometric exercises should be limited.

142. C: If a patient is admitted to the ED and reports no relief of chest pain after taking nitroglycerine three times at 5-minute intervals and the presumptive diagnosis is unstable angina or NSTEMI, the initial treatment should include oxygen and the antiplatelet agent ASA. If the patient cannot tolerate ASA, then clopidogrel may be substituted. ECG monitoring and intravenous access should be started, and the patient should be further evaluated to determine whether conservative or invasive management is indicated.

143. A: The ECG findings that most suggest coronary ischemia are ST-segment depression at least 1 mm below isoelectric line (the flat line that occurs when no electrical impulse is being recorded) and T-wave inversion. As damage to the myocardium occurs, the ST-segment elevates with elevation ≥1 mm above the isoelectric line significant. Prompt treatment of cardiac injury may prevent infarction, and this can be confirmed with cardiac markers. Pathologic Q waves may occur with myocardial infarction, usually indicating that at least 50% of the thickness of the myocardium is affected.

144. B: A dysrhythmia characterized by a regular heart rate of 160 beats per minute with abnormally shaped P waves (that may be hidden in the preceding T waves) but with a normal PR interval and normal QRS complex is paroxysmal supraventricular tachycardia. The electrical discharge can originate anywhere above the bifurcation of the bundle of His. Onset is usually abrupt, and termination may be followed by a brief asystole. Some degree of AV block is also commonly observed.

145. D: The cardiac/vascular nurse would expect a patient being admitted for acute decompensated heart failure to present with pulmonary edema. Typically, the patient will be pale, anxious, cold, and clammy, and they may appear cyanotic. Respiratory rate is usually more than 30 per minute, and the patient usually feels severely dyspneic and exhibits orthopnea. Tachycardia is often present, and BP may be elevated or reduced, depending on the patient's condition. Crackles, rales, and rhonchi may be noted throughout the lung fields.

146. A: A pacemaker with the NBG code of VDD senses both atria and ventricles but paces only ventricles. Pacemakers and ICDs are assigned three to five letter codes. The NBG code is:

(1) Paced chambers	(2) Sensed chambers	(3) Response mode	(4) Programmable features	(5) Anti-tachycardic features
V-ventricle A-atrium D-dual O-none	V-ventricle A-atrium D-dual O-none	T-triggered I-inhibited D-dual O-none	R-rate modulated C-communicating M-multiprogrammable P-simple programmable O-none	O-none P-paced S-shocks D-dual

147. C: Following radiofrequency ablation, the patient must be taught to monitor the pulse daily and note any indications of arrhythmias, keeping a record for the physician, because arrhythmias may recur. Patients should be taught to look for any signs of infection around the catheter insertion site, such as drainage, erythema, or pain, and should be reminded of the importance of taking the full course of prophylactic antibiotics, which may need to be taken for up to 12 weeks.

148. C: If a patient's functional capacity allows for medium activity (3.5–5.0 METS), the work activity that is allowable is mowing lawns.

METS	Activity
1.5–2.5	Driving, typing, sewing, walking 2 mph, desk work, doing light carpentry, carrying 15–30 lb
2.5–3.5	Using hand tools, woodworking, house painting
3.5–5.0	Gardening, making beds, moving lawns
5–7	Using pneumatic tools, plumbing, carrying 30–60 lb
7–9	Shoveling, digging ditches, carrying 60–90 lb
Over 9	Heavy, strenuous activities, carrying over 90 lb

149. D: According to Tong's criteria for decision-making in relation to the principle of justice, the criterion that has priority is need. Determining who receives priority can pose ethical dilemmas, especially when care is determined by the ability to pay—a common finding in healthcare because of inequities in healthcare coverage. Criteria related to justice include providing to each according to:

1. Equal share
2. Need
3. Effort
4. Contribution
5. Merit
6. Ability to pay

150. A: The second heart sound, S2, may exhibit splitting:

- Physiological: occurs on inspiration when an increased volume of blood returns to the right side of the heart and a decreased amount to the left because of the expanded lung trapping blood
- Pathological: occurs on both inspiration and expiration
- Paradoxical: occurs when anything causes late closure of the aortic valve (such as electrical delay caused by left bundle branch), mechanical obstruction (aortic stenosis), or impaired left ventricular function

It's Your Moment, Let's Celebrate It!

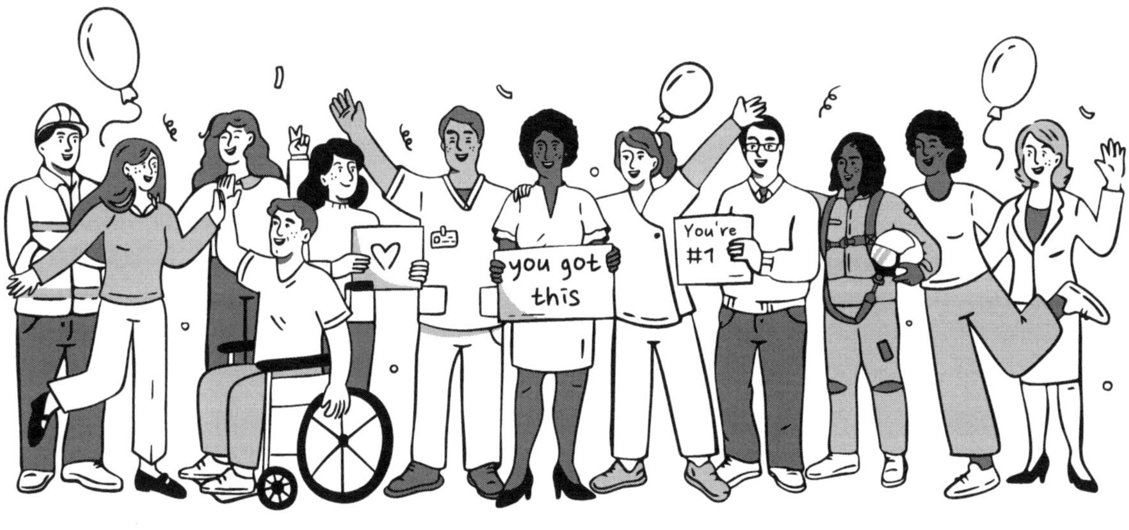

Share your story @mometrixtestpreparation